M000191241

INDECENT

**How I Make It
and Fake It
as a Girl For Hire**

Sarah Katherine Lewis

SEAL PRESS

INDECENT
How I Make It and Fake It as a Girl for Hire
Copyright © 2006 Sarah Katherine Lewis

Published by Seal Press
An Imprint of Avalon Publishing Group, Incorporated
1400 65th Street, Suite 250
Emeryville, CA 94608

All rights reserved. No part of this book may be reproduced or transmitted in any form without written permission from the publisher, except by reviewers who may quote brief excerpts in connection with a review.

ISBN-13: 978-1-58005-169-9
ISBN-10: 1-58005-169-3

9 8 7 6 5 4 3 2

Library of Congress Cataloging-in-Publication Data

Lewis, Sarah Katherine.
Indecent : how I make it and fake it as a girl for hire / Sarah Katherine Lewis.
p. cm.
ISBN-13: 978-1-58005-169-9
ISBN-10: 1-58005-169-3
1. Pornography—United States. 2. Sex-oriented businesses—United States. I. Title.
HQ472.U6L48 2006
306.770973--dc22
    2006012045

Cover design by Patrick David Barber
Interior design by Tabitha Lahr
Printed in the United States of America by Malloy
Distributed by Publishers Group West

The author has changed some names, places, and identifying details in this book to protect the privacy of individuals.

This book is dedicated to the working ladies of Seattle, Washington, of course—the smartest, funniest, kindest, wisest, and most beautiful women in the entire world.

This book is also dedicated to my teacher, Mr. Lyall Bush, the executive director of Richard Hugo House. Thank you for your astonishing brilliance, your kindness, and your giddy passion for good writing. Hemingway still sucks, though.

Contents

Introduction
Floor Show

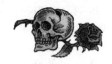

"Set It Off" — Peaches

When I was very young, I saw a woman behind glass on a cop show on TV. She was being questioned by one of the show's detectives, and in order to interrogate her through the glass, he had to put a few dollars into a machine that lifted the curtain between the two of them. As he demanded answers from the woman, she casually lifted her feet—spreading her legs—and hooked her heels at the top of the glass window, treating the embarrassed detective to a panoramic and frankly gynecological view of her privates. Of course they couldn't show this on TV—the camera angled behind the detective so all you could see was his back, not the woman's vagina. The detective was completely unmanned by her display. His confident questions devolved into broken half sentences and he stared at the floor, blushing instead of gazing at what the woman was so contentedly flaunting.

I can't remember how the cop show turned out, but I'll never forget my rapture at the idea of working behind glass, and the woman's insouciant use of her own body to shock and provoke. I figured that woman had the absolute best job in the world. She was safe behind glass, without anyone telling her what to do! And when men put money in to lift the curtain, all she had to do was show them her body. When they were done looking at it, she could read and wait for the next customer. The scenario was both erotic and practical. At nine, I imagined myself in a glass box, spreading my legs challengingly, my book temporarily set aside. *If you could work in a glass cube,* I thought, *why on earth* wouldn't *you?*

At the same time I knew better than to tell my politically liberal, college-educated parents about my new obsession. Being behind glass—showing men my body for money—was not only dirty, it was *unfeminist,* like wanting to be a bride or a stay-at-home mom or a *Playboy* model. It was *bad for women.* It was *exploitative.* Women who did that kind of thing were misguided tools, pitiable playthings for men—they were throwing their lives away and actively collaborating with the kind of villians who conspired to defeat the ERA, over and over again.

In private, my friends and I played a game called Whore. We took turns dressing up and being the whore, which meant standing with one hip cocked and displaying a tough, bemused sneer. We'd ask each other, "Want a date?" to which the expected response was, "How much?" None of us knew how much, though, and none of us were sure what to do after the initial verbal exchange. Still, we loved playing Whore and did so whenever we were certain we wouldn't be interrupted by our parents. We knew we would have been busted big-time for our game—even saying the word *whore* was risky. We referred to Whore as "The Game" in shameful, excited whispers.

When I was sixteen, instead of becoming a whore, I got my first job—working behind the counter at a bagel bakery. Soon after that I learned to make espresso and embarked upon a career predicated on ristretto shots and light, perfectly frothed cappuccino foam. Eventually I graduated from high school and started waiting tables at a local "bistro"—really just a neighborhood joint with French pretensions, featuring overpriced, undercooked slabs of halibut and a thirteen-dollar beef stew that was mostly potatoes. When I got sick of waitressing, I went back to making coffee.

And so it went: I ricocheted between table service and counter service, working full-time but never making enough to do more than make ends meet. Some months the ends refused to meet no matter how many extra shifts I begged for. I learned to guzzle milk on the sly, and to eat food from the half-eaten plates I retrieved from my tables.

At twenty-four, I was unemployed, after having been fired from a local corporate coffee franchise for "insubordination." I was sick of making coffee anyway—sick of smiling at rude customers, sick of being controlled by management in every respect, from my bathroom breaks to my choice of attire.

I considered myself a feminist. Why not? I'd done all the reading, exhausting the women's studies section of the downtown Seattle Public Library, from Betty Friedan to Andrea Dworkin to Simone de Beauvoir. Consequently I was very aware of the new school of thought about sex work—that it was "empowering" and "transgressive"; that women could choose to do it from a powerful, self-determined stance instead of being passive victims in a system that didn't respect their needs. I was intrigued. I knew all about being a passive victim in a system that didn't respect my needs—I'd been working in food service for over eight years.

Sex work—whatever that was—had to be better than food service; I was sure of that. And now it was okay for feminists to do it! My secret obsession, the game of Whore—recast as an assertive, feminist act! I'd never forgotten the woman in the glass booth, spreading her legs and showing herself to the detective—turning the tables on him in one outrageous fuck-you gesture. I could do that! I wanted a chance to feel that powerful, that strong! I could handle being objectified—could even *enjoy* being objectified—as long as I was making money and calling all the shots. Right?

The Lusty Lady had women behind glass, I knew—but their ads made it sound like you had to be a fashion model to work there. And as much as I ached to fulfill my childhood fantasy, I lacked the confidence to even apply. I was pretty sure no strip club would hire me, either—I was stocky, with no dance training.

But I was determined to find something—*some* venue—where I could cock one hip saucily and ask, "Want a date?" and still be a feminist; where I could read between clients and make men stammer and turn red at will. I knew there had to be a place for me somewhere. I just had to find it.

Chapter 1
Jack Shack

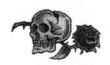

"Do Ya Think I'm Sexy?" — The Revolting Cocks

Butterscotch's Live Lingerie Adult Tanning was a rundown little storefront about half a mile from my equally rundown little apartment.

I had no idea what a Live Lingerie Adult Tan was. I thought that perhaps Butterscotch's was a tanning salon that featured a lingerie-clad staff—like Hooters, but without the hula hoops and chicken wings.

I had to be honest with myself, though: There was something unsavory about Butterscotch's. I never saw anyone go in or come out from the front door, and it stayed open late, like a tattoo parlor or a bar. The shades were always down, even in the middle of the afternoon, and the neon sign looked gaudy and kind of—adult, I supposed; like a strip club. The sign showed a blond, faceless woman in a corset and high heels, with the word "Butterscotch's" underneath her in flowing cursive script. I supposed that if you were trying to encourage men to tan by promising Live Lingerie— whatever that was—advertising your business with the image of a sexy lady was only smart.

As I entered the lobby and heard the door buzzer go off, *beep beep beeeeeeep,* like a fire alarm, I was smacked in the face by a thick cloud of funk. The stink was a deep and multilayered construction: Dueling top notes of Lysol and vomitously sweet vanilla-scented air freshener just barely covered the rich stench of human bodies and mildew, and underneath that, the powdery reek of baby oil provided a nostril-curling finish. It was hot and stuffy in the lobby, like someone had turned the heat up as far as it would go and then just forgot about it. I didn't want to touch anything. It was hard to breathe, and I immediately started sweating.

I noticed a camera behind the desk pointed right at me, the little red light blinking, and felt exposed. I wanted to act normal but I had no idea *how*, or what kind of behavior was appropriate. Should I act casual? Professional? Shady and embarrassed, the way I imagined people acted in strip clubs? *But this isn't a strip club*, I reminded myself. It was a tanning salon of some sort—with lingerie, somehow, but still—a legitimate business, offering professional skin damage as a legitimate service. I wasn't here to gawk at women in corsets and heels—I was here to get a job being one of them.

I sat down in a battered chair near the desk, next to a glass-topped coffee table covered in ragged magazines. I crossed my legs and attempted to leaf through a magazine, until I realized it was covered in baby oil. Dropping it back on the pile, I wiped my hands on my pants. *Ugh.*

My eyes gradually adjusted to the weird gloom of the lobby. I gazed around in increasing dismay.

The interior of Butterscotch's was grimy and trollish; everything was dirty and abandoned looking. The furnishings were either half-assedly repaired or just left broken. Half the fluorescent light panel was out, and the other half fluttered on and off. I tried to breathe deeply, but the thick, bad-smelling air made me feel worse, not better.

The broken-slatted plastic blinds over the front window were covered in dust and repaired with duct tape. Dead, dried-up gnats dusted the sills like fresh-ground pepper. The neon sign buzzed and flickered, connected to its outlet by a series of jerry-rigged extension cords that stretched across the room over the threadbare carpet, like a trip wire. One of the cords was wrapped in duct tape, too. Another glass coffee table supported a display of tanning products—all different sizes of bottles and brands, every single one dusty and haphazardly arranged. Some of the bottles looked like they'd been opened.

Butterscotch's didn't look like a business to me. It looked like some junkie's apartment. All the lobby needed to complete the illusion was a hotplate and a sad, neglected cat box overflowing with fossilized shit.

I got up to go, but as I stood, a door behind the desk opened, and a really short girl in the highest heels I'd ever seen walked out. Her gait was weird, like she wasn't used to her shoes or maybe she'd just put them on. She was wearing a blue velvet minidress. I thought flats would have been a better choice, since the hem of the skirt was just under her ass and everyone knows the shorter the skirt, the flatter the heel. Her face was so beautiful I couldn't really take it in all at once: She had black bangs like Bettie Page, and long silky hair, and she wore black liquid eyeliner across her upper lids, and I had honestly never seen a woman look the way she did except in magazines. Her skin was so porcelain-smooth she looked like she'd been airbrushed.

Suddenly, I was ashamed of myself. The lobby may have been dank and grimy, but this girl was beautiful, and beautiful girls always made me feel embarrassed and tongue-tied. My face felt hot. Who was I trying to kid? There was no way I could ever, ever look like that. And if that was the standard for employment, I felt like asking for an application would just be embarrassing for both of us.

"Hi," she said, smiling as graciously as a society hostess. "Are you here to apply?" She sat behind the desk, her legs crossed high.

Did men fall in love with her instantly? I wondered if old foreign men stopped her and said stuff in their native tongues like *Your eyes are as blue as the Old Country's skies!* and got teary and maybe even crossed themselves or blessed her in some way. For some reason, I pictured these men in billowy white shirts, wearing little newsboys' caps and maybe embroidered vests, like organ grinders.

In that moment, I realized I wanted to work at Butterscotch's so badly I could feel my desire as a physical craving. The scary, squalid lobby didn't even matter. Whatever this girl had—whatever made her so perfect, so self-possessed and cool and amazing—I wanted it, with all my heart. Those glossy lips, and those swooping black eyebrows, as arched as an old movie star's! I could never be her. Never. But if I could work with her, maybe I could—watch her? Learn from her? I didn't know. I felt dizzy, delirious with need.

"Yeah, I'm here to . . ." All of a sudden I just couldn't stand it. "Okay, listen, am I too fat to work here?" I asked.

"No! No way," the Bettie Page girl said. She seemed like she was being honest, and was sincerely surprised at my question. "Well, I mean, stand up."

I did, and put my hands out. I turned around slowly, sucking in my gut, and kind of tucking my butt in and under, like a dog hiding its tail. I was trying to look as unfat as I possibly could. I felt huge. She was so tiny, like a pretty little doll.

"No, you're totally fine," she said. "Nice tits."

"*Really?*" My heart was pounding. *She likes me! She likes my tits!* I felt like punching the air in triumphant joy. I was glad I'd worn my tightest tank top.

"Okay, then, how do I apply?"

She rummaged in the desk, and handed me a xeroxed application. "Fill this out and bring it back," she said. "The manager is Crystal. She'll like you." She paused. "I'm Lenore."

"Oh, that's pretty! I love that name! Wasn't there a Lenore in Poe? Though, am I thinking of Hawthorne?" I wanted to slap myself to stop my insipid slurry of words.

Lenore laughed—a low purr, nice and tasteful, like a lady at a cocktail party. It sounded like clinking ice and expensive liquor. She didn't answer. Her back was so straight. She was like a ballet dancer or something, just sitting in the busted old office chair, looking comfortable and elegant.

"I'll bring this back tomorrow. Th—thank you." Stuttering! I wanted to die.

I just knew Lenore was thinking about what a big, fat, inept asshole I was. I imagined her at a small, chic soiree in her blue velvet dress, sipping her drink and telling the story of the stuttering fat girl who wanted to work as a lingerie-wearing tanning salon model. I saw her surrounded by admiring men, all laughing and listening to her soft, sophisticated alto. "And then she ran out the door, boys," Lenore was saying, batting lush black eyelashes like Scarlett O'Hara. "And I never saw her giant posterior, ever again!" More laughing, and the tinkly sounds of jazz piano in the background.

I still didn't even know how the tanning fit in, or what the job was, exactly. The whole time I'd been there, the phone hadn't rung, and no customers had gone in or come out. Why was the lobby so shabby, and why was Lenore so breathtaking? How in the world did those two things go together? Could I possibly be like Lenore, if I bought a cocktail dress and high-heeled shoes and learned how to do my makeup like some vintage movie star's? Was the potential there?

I thought that maybe—just maybe—the potential *was* there. After all, I was tall. I had a fat *posterior*, true, but I also had a small waist. And I definitely had nice tits—Lenore had said so! I could learn. I could fake it. I could just laugh and not answer people, and people would think I was cool and smooth and mysterious. Furthermore, I could change my laugh from loud and embarrassing to soft and silky. Like Lenore's.

As I walked home I thought about Butterscotch's. Was it really a viable business? Where did the actual tanning come into play? Why was the lobby so awful? Were all the girls who worked there as exquisite as Lenore? So many things didn't match: The dead bugs on the windowsills didn't go with Lenore's expertly applied lip liner. The grime on the wall and the sad, tampered-with tanning products didn't jibe with her graceful posture. The buzzing sign, and most of all the *smell*, that horrible sickening filthy reek, didn't match up with Lenore's elegance and glamour. It was like she didn't even smell the place, or like she existed on some kind of physical plane on which all bad smells magically changed into the smell of tea roses.

That evening I bought liquid eyeliner at the drugstore and spent hours in front of my bathroom mirror trying to apply it close to my lash line without smearing. It was incredibly frustrating. I couldn't figure out how Lenore did it. I could get one eye done nicely, but getting the other one to match it was impossible. As hard as I tried, I'd either poke myself in the eye with the little brush or end up painting the liner a quarter inch above my actual eyelashes. I looked like a crazy, homeless old lady—all I needed was coral lipstick, rubbed loonily over my mouth and teeth.

After I washed all the black liner off, rubbing my eyes red with a washcloth, I looked over the Butterscotch's application. After the standard *Name, Address, Phone Number,* and *Last Three Jobs* crap, there was an instruction: *Describe yourself in three words.*

I put *Smart.* Then I crossed that out and wrote *Confident.* Then I felt like an idiot, put Wite-Out over both words, and wrote, *Sophisticated. Elegant. Ladylike.*

I figured that's what Lenore would have written. I needed a rubber bracelet with WHAT WOULD LENORE DO? printed on it, like those Jesus bracelets, that I could snap when I needed to concentrate.

The next question: *What's your favorite part of your body?*

Torso, I wrote. *Tits.* I whited out *tits,* and replaced it with *breasts.* Then I whited out *breasts.* I thought that mentioning them might be indiscreet.

Height? Five foot eight.

Weight? I paused. *150 pounds,* I wrote slowly. It looked like a lie. It was written in too carefully, like I was choosing my words, instead of just dashing them off spontaneously. True, I *was* lying—I really weighed about 160. I wore a size 12/14, and my build was usually referred to kindly as *statuesque* by well-meaning apologists. To mitigate the lie of my weight, I hastily added, *Curvy build—36D.* Fuck discretion.

Then I went back, whited out my height, and made it *five foot nine.*

Why do you want to work here? was the last question on the application.

Dear Crystal, I wrote. *I would like to be a member of the Butterscotch's team. I am a team player and very easy to get along with. I think I would be a valuable asset to your staff. I am a hard worker, and I give every professional challenge my all.*

I wasn't sure if I was on the right track. WWLD?

I am confident in my allure and would be delighted to share my love of fine lingerie and excellent customer service, as a representative of a reputable establishment like Butterscotch's Live Lingerie Adult Tanning. Thank you very much for your consideration. References available upon request.

It's hard to apply for jobs when you're not exactly sure what they are. I signed the application, wrote my preferred model name in the blank—"Emma," for Emma Goldman—and went to bed.

"Strangers on a Train"— Lovage

A few days after I returned my application to Butterscotch's, I got a call from Crystal. She sounded young and businesslike. "Lenore's taking a few days off to go down to L.A.," she said. "Can you come in for training today at three? And then plan to stay until midnight for your first shift?"

"Yes, ma'am," I said. "Absolutely!"

"Bring a non-see-through bra, a thong—*not* a G-string—a pair of shoes, and something to cover yourself up with, like a slip or a short robe. Also, a short dress or miniskirt set to wear in the lobby." I thought of Lenore's blue dress with longing. I didn't own anything that pretty.

"A thong, not a G-string?" I felt like an idiot. "Aren't they the same thing?"

"No," Crystal sighed. "You've never done this before? Shit.

"A G-string is with the string in the back. A thong has at least one inch of fabric. We aren't allowed to wear G-strings because they show too much pink. Make sure your thong covers all your pink parts, isn't see-through or made of lace, and is at least one inch wide in the back. Okay?"

I couldn't believe the whole "pink parts" thing. It was like when Lenore said *tits*. I had no response; I was blushing too hard.

15

I had never worn any panties in my life that hadn't completely covered not only my "pink parts," but also my entire ass. The nasty thong panties they sold as sets with push-up bras—the ones cut to go between the wearer's butt cheeks—had always seemed like the visual equivalent of dirty jokes to me: similar to the inflatable plastic sheep sold for bachelor parties, or those cupcakes topped with body parts made of hard, sugary frosting. I didn't realize that anyone would actually *wear* them, any more than they'd parade around in those Fruit Leathery edible panties that adult novelty stores sell next to the plastic blow-up sheep and the banana-shaped dildos. I wasn't even sure where to go to get thong panties, or if they even came in my size. Plus, didn't the strip in the back rub up against your actual ass*hole*? Was that even hygienic?

"Okay?" asked Crystal. "Any questions?"

"Uh, no," I said. "I'll see you at three. And thank you very much."

"You're welcome," Crystal said. She sounded bemused.

It was noon. I had three hours. I needed to go shopping.

But first I took a long, uncomfortably hot bath. I scrubbed my asshole with Ivory soap and a washcloth, vigorously, until I felt a little sore. I put on a pair of white cotton bikini panties, and they felt soft and good against my skin.

I had twelve identical pairs of white cotton panties in my underwear drawer that I'd bought in two plastic-sealed six-packs. It had never occurred to me to buy any other colors or styles. I just wore them, washed them, and put them back in my drawer to be worn again. Of course they were a little baggy, and tended to ride low on my hips. But they were just panties. Who cared about panties? They were just something to wear—necessary items, like socks.

The shiny panties made out of cheap satin, sold from bins instead of in sensible plastic packages—the ones with designs and sassy slogans—I never knew who bought those. I kind of thought maybe they were just jokes. They always looked so small when I held them up between pinched fingers—tiny triangles of shoddy fabric connected by complicated strips or tied strings. I usually had a hard time telling which part was supposed to go in front.

I put a tank top in my backpack, and added a short, elastic-waisted skirt I'd always hated. I figured I could wear that in the lobby of Butterscotch's until I figured out where to go to buy a dress like Lenore's. I didn't have a slip or a robe, so after deliberating, I added a man's suit jacket to my pack. It was kind of boxy, with thin lapels—I'd bought it secondhand and it had been cheap, because the matching trousers were missing—and I figured it might look kind of hot with lingerie under it. I imagined myself as Sally Bowles, vamping on a stool with a hat tipped over one eye.

Victoria's Secret was the only place I knew to go for underwear besides places like Sears. I took the bus to the one downtown, where I bought a plain black bra, a matching thong, and some thigh-high stockings. Then I went to Payless and bought a pair of chunky, high-heeled shoes, with straps across the instep to keep them on. I tried them on, couldn't walk, and hoped I'd get used to them. Finally, I went to the drugstore and bought a tube of Wet 'n' Wild lipstick—bright red.

I showed up to Butterscotch's half an hour early, with everything crammed into my pack except the shoes, which I carried.

The stench hit me as I walked in the door. It was sickening, like the world's worst case of BO crossed with urine, then sprayed with disinfectant. The heat made the reek even worse. It was like there was no air in Butterscotch's, only big, fluffy clouds of stink.

Beep beep beeeeeeeep went the buzzer. I stepped forward and stood in the middle of the lobby. "I'm here for an appointment with Crystal?" I said. "For training?" I heard giggling behind the door. Then, about a million years later, the door opened up and a tiny, washed-out blond woman stepped out to greet me.

She wore jeans—high-waisted, loose through the hips and thighs, and tapered at the ankles. They looked acid-washed, though it was hard to tell in the dim and flickering fluorescent light of the lobby. Her T-shirt had been cut off to expose her stomach, which was flat and lean. The shirt said TRAMP in a gothic font, like a tattoo. Her breasts hung low under her shirt—she clearly wasn't wearing a bra. She looked plain, normal—like any girl you'd see at the grocery store or out walking her dog around Green Lake. Her eyelashes were pale, giving her face a rabbity cast. She smiled at me.

"I'm Crystal," she said. "Are you Emma?"

"Yes," I said.

"Come on back."

I followed her through the door behind the desk.

The first thing I noticed was how dark it was. We were in a hall, but I couldn't see anything. Maybe some doors? The sweet reek of baby oil became even stronger. I heard a television, turned up loud. I followed Crystal's blond hair down the hall, up a short flight of stairs, and through a door.

We were in the room with the TV. A girl was stretched on a couch, watching the screen intently. She looked up—she was pretty, short-haired, Asian—said, "Hi," and returned her attention to her show. There was a pile of fashion magazines in the corner of the room, and a messy pile of blankets. A space heater was on, making the room sauna-hot. Which made sense, because the Asian girl was in her bra and panties.

I blushed and looked away.

"This is the lounge," said Crystal. "This is Heather."

"Hi," I said.

"Heather, this is Emma. She's new."

Heather shrugged. The laugh track flared.

Crystal stepped back out of the room, into the pitch-black hall. I followed her to the room directly across from the lounge. "This is the dressing room," she said.

The room was shabby and small. A long makeup table held little grouped piles of cosmetics that I assumed belonged to the other girls. A mirror was lit with strings of Christmas tree lights, wrapped around and around it like a frame. Backpacks and piles of clothes were everywhere. Just off the dressing room was a tiny alcove containing a washer and a dryer. The room smelled of laundry detergent and mildew.

"Go ahead and change, and I'll give you the tour," said Crystal. She checked her watch: a big and mannish digital, strapped to her tiny wrist.

I expected her to leave, but Crystal just leaned up against the sagging makeup table and folded her arms.

I had never felt more obese in my life.

"Um, are you sure you want me to change right now? Maybe we should do the tour first?" I squeaked. I hated the way my voice trembled.

"Nah, go ahead," said Crystal. Her eyes were flat. "I have to see what you brought to wear, anyway."

My face felt frozen as I turned my back toward Crystal. Opening my pack and pulling out the pink-and-white striped Victoria's Secret bag seemed to take forever. My hands shook as I pulled the tags off each garment. I laid everything out. The black satin looked unbelievably sinister and slithery against the peeling shelf paper on the table. I couldn't believe I owned a thong. And that I was about to put it on.

In front of someone.

I unlaced my boots, took them off, took off my socks. Unbuckled my belt. Let my Levi's slide over my hips to the floor. Then I took my panties off. I tried to keep my thighs clamped together to hide my pussy. My pubic hair looked matted down and scruffy. I felt disgusting. I knew my cellulite showed in the bright fluorescent light. I was pretty sure Crystal was going to tell me to get dressed, get my stuff, and get out. *I made a horrible mistake*, I imagined her saying. And, *There's no way you're 150 pounds. You lied, you fat fuck!*

I tried to keep the side of my leg to Crystal so she couldn't see my puss or the rippled skin on the backs of my thighs. It was like trying to put on nylons over a chastity belt. I couldn't stop getting in my own way. Finally I got the thong on. It sat high over my hipbones, then plunged down in the middle, showing my navel. The one-inch strip of fabric in the back tucked itself between my ass cheeks, grazing my asshole. I felt unbelievably obscene.

"You gotta shave that," Crystal said.

"Excuse me?" I said. My puss? *Shave* it? Like a *porn star?* Were there special razors for that?

Crystal sighed.

"You have to shave your crotch," she said. "It's okay for today, just make sure all your crotch hair is tucked underneath your thong. You don't have much, anyway. But you have to be really careful about that: If you show hair, it's considered prostitution, and you can get arrested."

Arrested. Prostitution.

"And you gotta shave your armpits," she said.

I stared at her.

"This isn't France, hon," she said. "You're hired to be a fantasy girl. That means you have to look like a fantasy. Most men want smooth skin."

"I've—never shaved," I said. "Anything."

Crystal looked at me like I was insane. "And wear deodorant," she said slowly.

It occurred to me that I had absolutely no idea of what I was doing. I didn't wear deodorant, or shave, or wear high heels. I'd always known that some women did, but I thought those women were the exceptions—nasty little Barbie dolls, prissy and stuck-up and somehow dirty. Fake. I didn't know any women who bought razors, or wore thongs. I had thought that most women were like me.

True, my body hair was fine and light—but more than that, I had been raised to believe that feminists didn't fuss around with their natural appearances, and that deodorant was unnecessary if you used soap and water every day. Considering the alternative opened up whole worlds of anxiety. Would I be expected to shave my legs every day? Would Crystal line us up and check our skin for smoothness? And a shaved crotch—I wasn't even sure how you'd do that without help. Though I had to admit there was something insidiously sexy and luxurious about the idea of being so bare down there. It seemed so *dirty*—not just naughty, but excitingly depraved. I felt a small quiver of anticipation.

I finished dressing, rolling the stockings up my legs and immediately snagging one. Great. They'd cost $12, more than I'd ever paid for tights. The elastic waist of the skirt cut into my skin.

At least my tits look good, I thought, feeling a little sexy as I looked at myself—half-dressed and red-faced—in the mirror. The bra held them up nicely, presenting them like two scoops of vanilla ice cream on a tray. I thought the bra made me look kind of Lenoreish, kind of vintagey. If only I had a slinky cocktail dress to wear over my new bra and panties, instead of my stupid tank top and skirt!

In my new Payless shoes, I towered over Crystal. "You need to get higher heels," she said. "With a stiletto heel."

"Okay," I said. *Higher* heels? I could barely walk on the heels I was wearing.

"You can do your makeup later. I have to get going at four, so let's do the tour," said Crystal.

"Okay." I staggered after her, sliding my feet on the carpet and using my hand covertly against the wall to stay steady and upright.

We passed the lounge, went down the stairs, and were in the pitch-black hall again.

"Are we going to the tanning beds?" I asked.

Crystal laughed.

"Fire Woman" — The Cult

We were in a tiny room, like a veal pen. A nearly identical room was next door—Crystal had showed it to me. Our room was slightly bigger, which is why we were in it. I sat on a white bath towel, on a couch. The room was lit by a dim lamp, which sat on a coffee table to the right of the couch. The lamp shared the table with a bottle of baby oil, some dog-eared copies of *Maxim* and *Stuff,* and a pile of folded washcloths. There was a metal chair in front of me.

The room smelled strongly of bleach, air freshener, and baby oil—like the lobby of Butterscotch's, but somehow more *intimate.* More private. I kept thinking it smelled like sweat, or old clothes, but neither of those things was right. It smelled like someone's bedroom, or someone's bathroom, or a locker room. It stank the way some people stink—a specific funk of unhealth, covered up with acrid, perfumy chemical esters. I was conscious of the feel of the towel beneath the bare skin of my ass cheeks. I wasn't used to that skin being touched by anything but white cotton. The inch of fabric against my asshole rubbed a little as I shifted on the towel.

I pulled at the snag in my stocking with my thumbnail, turning it into a long nylon ladder running the length of my thigh.

Crystal had changed out of her jeans and T-shirt and into a white bra, matching thong panties, a lacy slip, and high platform shoes. The shoes were made of see-through plastic and had clear pointy heels with little air bubbles suspended in them. I had never seen shoes like them before. Even though the clear plastic had yellowed a little, it was exciting to be able to see her entire foot, right through the shoes. Her feet were arched like the feet on the Barbies I'd owned when I was little, and her toenails were red and chipped. She walked confidently in her plastic heels, picking her feet up off the carpet quickly and putting them back down again, like a show pony. Her ankles looked thin, as if they might break at any moment.

Kneeling, Crystal slipped a CD into the boom box that sat on the floor near a standing triptych of mirrors. The glass of the mirrors was smoky, and there were little streaks of gold painted on them. They looked like they belonged in the bathroom of someone who wore too much cologne and a lot of gold chains.

Mirrors also lined one side of the room. You could see endless Crystals reflected back and forth between the mirrored wall and the standing mirrors. You could see her back and her front at the same time as the music started playing and she stood up.

She approached me, smiling. Tossed her long, pale hair around. Shook it like a curtain.

Running her hands along the sides of her body, she gently cupped her breasts, showing their shape to me. Coyly, she stepped closer in those plastic shoes, turning and displaying her bottom under the lacy slip. She kicked one leg up gracefully, and I noticed how smooth and pretty her skin was. I guess she probably shaved. The way she moved around and shimmied, it was like she was prancing. She was in time with the music, but she wasn't dancing, exactly. Rather she was showing off the prettiest parts of her body to me, over and over, in different ways.

And she wasn't my type of girl, not at all, but I couldn't take my eyes off her. I just couldn't. I had never seen anything like her performance before, had never known that anything like it could even exist.

The first song ended as she shed her slip, letting it fall to the floor and then stepping out of it daintily. She smiled at me again. I thought of the word *seductive*. I was frozen.

In her white bra and thong, she was child-size and hairless. I looked between her legs, and it seemed like she was smooth in front—sealed, like a doll, no vulva or lips to interrupt the silky sweep of her panties. I couldn't imagine piss coming from there, or blood, or anything.

Crystal came close to me and I smelled her skin, light and soapy, like flowers. She shook her hair again and I could smell that, too. Then, slipping her shoes off, she leapt up lightly onto the couch. Straddling my face, tiny legs spread. Not touching.

She rotated her little hips, cocking them saucily like a burlesque dancer. It was sexy, but it was also *cute*. I kept thinking of Tinkerbell, in her little jagged-hemmed dress, and even though she was mostly naked, was Tinkerbell *nasty?* No. She was almost sexless, despite her undeniably feminine build. Crystal was like that: so little, so cute, and even when she went backward on her hands on the metal chair—spreading her legs so I could see the entire uninterrupted strip of fabric that went between her legs, an inch of satin covering her vagina and her anus—she was like a pixie, levitating and swirling and hopping around, as if she weighed less than the hot, stuffy air around her.

I had never been so close to a woman I wasn't making love to.

I had never seen a woman's body that *little,* and that smooth. I'd never seen a pussy, hiding behind satin, that looked like it didn't even have an opening, let alone lips or a protruding clitoral hood. All the pussies I'd ever licked or fucked had been hairy, and had lovely, luscious, oysterish scents. Those pussies had distinct, lovable *personalities,* as individual and fierce and earthy as the women they belonged to. Those pussies were forces of nature, between strong, thick, beautiful thighs.

This pussy, on the other hand, was *sanitized.* It was ethereal. I couldn't imagine doing anything with it.

I couldn't breathe.

"Crystal—" I said. Then I couldn't say anything.

The third song started. Crystal hopped down from the couch and knelt between my knees, pushing the chair back expertly, without even looking at it.

I was embarrassed to be so big, with my legs spread open. Could she smell me? Had I washed enough? I inadvertently tightened my thighs, but I couldn't close them because Crystal was right there in between them.

Crystal shook her hair forward, until it was draped across the top of my stocking. I could feel her breath against the front of my panties. It made me feel like I had to pee, or scream. She looked up at me from between the Y of my thighs, made sure I was looking at her, and began—I guess the word is *fellating*—her own index finger.

My face felt like it was going to crack into shards. I watched. I couldn't do anything else.

I became conscious of a throb between my legs.

I thought, *If I had a penis, I'd want to put it inside every woman I saw.*

I watched her painted nail disappear between her lips, over and over again. She licked like a kitten, showing sharp little teeth. Finally, she moved her wet and glistening finger out of her mouth, trailed it down her swannish neck, and rubbed it between her breasts, using her skinny upper arms to push them together for a surprisingly cavernous cleavage.

The song ended. Crystal stood up briskly, wiping her finger against her hip to dry it.

"So yeah, basically you just kind of do that," she said. "Act sexy for three songs, and if they need a little bit of extra time, maybe give them one more short song to finish up."

"Extra time?" I asked. "You mean, if they ask to see more?"

Crystal stared at me. "No," she said, slowly. "You don't need to show them any more. You never take off your bra or thong. *Ever.*"

She paused. "And never, ever touch them, or let them touch you. You notice how I never touched you?"

"Your hair," I said. "It touched my—leg." I blushed. Hard.

"Hair is legal," she said, simply. "Remember, no nipples, no flashing, no pubic hair or pink parts visible, *ever*. No touching, *ever*."

"Crystal," I said. "When you said 'finish up' . . . ?"

"Yeah?"

"What are they finishing? How do you know they're finished? Do they just kind of look away, or something?" Did they pick up one of the beat-up magazines on the coffee table and began leafing through it discreetly?

Crystal sighed.

"Most of them are nude, and they're—" She made a loose-wristed sliding gesture. "You can tell they're done when they come."

"I'm sorry?"

"They *masturbate*," said Crystal. "The show is over when they *come*."

I laughed nervously. I laughed till I started coughing.

I'd slept with men, sure. But I'd never seen a hard cock in action before. I mean, sex with men normally happened so fast—one minute you're kissing, the next minute you feel them all hard up against you, then they're inside you. There isn't a lot of time to stop and stare, like it's some kind of nature show. Then a few minutes later it's over, and you're back to normal again. At that point, it would be rude to look, wouldn't it? So I never had. Sex was awkward enough without the staring anyway.

As for men masturbating, I wasn't really sure what they did. I thought that a guy would maybe just make a fist and squeeze it around his cock, like his fist was a vagina or something. Maybe he'd put baby oil in the fist first to make it wet, like a pussy.

"Are you serious?" I giggled. "They just *do* that, right in front of us? Like they're peeing?" I couldn't believe it. "Aren't they *shy?*"

Crystal stared at me.

"Be sure they use the washcloth," she said. "No pointing their stuff at you."

I nodded. The whole thing seemed so insane. Who would actually *do* this?

"Any questions?"

I did have one, actually.

"Where are the tanning beds?"

She laughed. "There's one bed in the back. I'll show you. Most customers don't bother, though."

"But isn't that—?"

Crystal sighed.

"2Wicky"— Hooverphonic

After we finished in the veal pen, or the "showroom," as Crystal called it (which made it sound to me like we sold cars or major appliances), she walked me over to the tanning room. It contained one scratched and dented Wolff tanning bed, a broken chair, and some cardboard boxes, haphazardly stacked against one wall.

Crystal showed me how to use little yellow drop envelopes to pay the house for each session. We weren't paid by the hour; we were independent contractors, paid per show. The customers gave us $60 or $80, depending on if they wanted a basic lingerie show or a fetish show, and out of that we gave the house $40. We kept all our own tips. We had to fill out the little yellow envelopes correctly, or it would look like we were stealing. Girls who stole were fired immediately.

"Fetish shows are like if the customer wants you to talk dirty, or if he wants a session in the dungeon, or if he wants you to wear something special," said Crystal. "Shit, I have to go. Have I showed you the dungeon yet?"

"No," I said. We walked to the end of the hall, across from the bathroom the models shared with the customers. The dungeon turned out to be another veal pen, but painted black, with fewer mirrors and no couch and a big metal cage in the corner. Black leather riding crops and floggers hung from hooks on the wall, and baskets full of clothespins and plain white wax candles sat on a small table. In one corner of the room was a freestanding wooden cross with shackles hanging from the horizontal beam. The cross was covered with blobs of melted white wax that looked like bird droppings.

"Ta-da," said Crystal. "You won't be doing fetish shows for a while, but ask me or Viva or Lenore if you want to learn how to do domination later."

"Okay," I said. I actually felt pretty comfortable with the idea of dominating men for money. The work seemed pretty stupid, but if a customer wanted to pay me to hit him with a paddle or listen to him call me "Mistress," I could do that, no problem. That actually seemed less weird than getting paid to dance around and watch him jerk off.

"Okay, I gotta go," said Crystal. "You can go hang out in the lounge with Heather till five. You'll be working with Viva tonight, actually. Just ask her if you have any questions. She's been here for a year, and she's really nice."

I said okay. I was getting used to how dark the hall was. I was even getting used to the smell—or maybe it just didn't smell as bad at the dungeon end of the hallway. We went back up the stairs. Crystal went into the dressing room to change back into her jeans and her TRAMP T-shirt, and I went into the lounge and sat on the couch next to Heather. We watched *The Fresh Prince of Bel-Air* together in silence.

Crystal stuck her head in the door. "Can you come in on Friday, for the morning shift?" she asked me. I noticed she was holding a motorcycle helmet.

I nodded. *Morning!* Who'd come to a place like this first thing in the morning? All I wanted in the morning was a strong pot of tea, not girls dancing around in their underwear.

"Okay, Emma. Have a good night! It'll be good to work with you." She smiled. Paused. "Uh, you need to paint your nails. Fingers and toes." She left.

A moment later, I heard the *beep beep beeeeeeeep* of the front door. Crystal was gone.

I looked over at Heather. She was pretty but not "fantasy girl" pretty, unless your fantasy is a short-haired skater girl with a few self-administered anarchy and Dead Kennedys tattoos on her arms. She had put a dress on over her lingerie and was curled up barefoot, eating carrots out of a Ziploc bag.

"Do you like working here?" I asked when the show went to a commercial for Pizza Hut. My stomach growled.

"Yeah," Heather said. "It's all right. I work here, then I go up to Hawaii to surf. When I'm out there I cook in a vegan restaurant, no stripping. But it's cool here. Everyone's nice."

"Thank you," I said. For what? *Idiot.*

During the next commercial I asked Heather, "How do the customers pick which girl they want?"

She looked at me, shocked. "They don't *pick.* We don't do cattle calls. We take turns going out to the lobby." She paused. "Didn't Crystal tell you that?"

"She was in a hurry, I think," I said.

Heather rolled her eyes. "Okay. When the dude comes in, whoever's up goes out to greet him. You say, 'Hi. What kind of show would you like?' and he'll say if he wants a regular or a fantasy show." She paused. "The fantasies are the dirty talk, or the dungeon, or cross-dressing, or whatever. Basically anything freaky. Those are eighty dollars."

"What if he doesn't like the girl who goes out?"

Heather looked at me. "You'll do fine," she said.

I felt like an ass. "No, but seriously," I said. "Do we just tell them to leave if they don't want the girl who's up?"

"No, just go get the other girl. It happens. But for real, you'll be fine." She paused. "Do you have anything else to wear, though?"

Fuck! "No," I said.

"Well, you'll be fine."

At ten minutes before five, Heather pulled on a pair of Dickies work pants and a T-shirt, threw her Ziploc bag of carrots into a backpack, and left. "Good luck," she said.

Beep beep beeeeeeeep.

I was alone—sitting on a couch in the lounge of Butterscotch's Live Lingerie Adult Tanning. Waiting for men to come in and give me money, to watch me take off my clothes and levitate like a pixie. Waiting to show strange men my brand-new thong panties.

Waiting to watch them masturbate into folded-up washcloths. Waiting to show them to the tanning room. Waiting to clean their body grease off the bed afterward.

I thought, *What the fuck am I doing here?*

I thought, *I could just leave.*

Instead I went into the dressing room and put on my Wet 'n' Wild lipstick. I couldn't get it exactly in the line of my lips, but I kind of smeared it around with my finger and made it look okay. I stared at myself. All I could see was the elastic on my skirt digging into my waist, making a roll of chub, and the run in my stocking, and the smeared lipstick that had stained one corner of my mouth.

Beep beep beeeeeeeep.

I froze.

I heard the door behind the desk opening. I called, "Hello . . . ?"

Silence. Then a girl appeared in the dressing room doorway. She frowned at me. Dropped a huge army duffel bag on the floor.

"Sorry I'm late," she muttered.

She used her forearm to sweep the counter clean of everyone else's makeup. The little bottles and palettes and tubes rained down onto the carpet. Some of the compacts and trays of eye shadow broke open, making little sandy areas of pigment in the shag. A lipstick rolled away forlornly, then stopped. "Stupid fucking bitches," she said. She used her army boot to kick the makeup out of her way, grinding her heels into the plastic cases. It was a makeup Armageddon. I grabbed my Wet 'n' Wild lipstick and concealed it in my fist. Was this girl crazy? She apparently hated makeup.

Or maybe it was just that she hated other girls' makeup.

Once the counter was clear, she opened her army pack and pulled out a plastic grocery sack filled with cosmetics. She carefully took each and every item out, lining them up against the mirror in order. I noticed she arranged the pots of eye shadow in a continuum, from the palest shade to the darkest. She had multiple pots of what appeared to be the exact same shade of brown. They were all opened and partially used.

"Do you mind?" the girl said.

I realized I'd been staring. "I'm sorry," I said.

Then, "Are you Viva?"

She frowned at me again. I didn't think she was going to answer, but eventually she hissed, "*Yes.*" Dismissing me, she turned to her cosmetics and made sure every single label was pointing forward.

Viva was terrifying. And beautiful. She was thin and long-boned like a model, with short, platinum blond dreadlocks. She didn't have any eyebrows at all. Her skin was a rich olive, smooth, like polished wood. Her upper lip curved sumptuously, set in a permanent sneer. She had scars on her face from piercings that had been taken out— one on her lower lip, and one on the side of her nostril.

Her ears were pointed at the top, like elf ears.

I finally understood the descriptive phrase *heart-shaped face.* Her cheekbones were broad and strong, making the top part of her face triangular, like a cat's. Her chin was small, with a feminine cleft. She didn't look like anyone I'd ever seen before—she didn't look like she was from here.

By "here," I didn't mean Seattle. I meant Earth.

Her eyes were all pupil, no iris. I wondered if she was on something. She seemed so angry. Her movements were fast and kind of jerky.

Beep . . . beep. Beeeeeeeeeep.

"Customer," said Viva.

I couldn't move.

Beeeeeeeeeeeeeep. Beep.

"Customer," she snarled. "Fuck! Are you gonna go, or what?"

"Yes," I said, slowly. I moved one foot, in its clunky horrible Payless shoe. Then I moved the other one. Clunk. I felt like my knees were fused: They wouldn't bend. I forced myself down the stairs, one hand splayed out on the wall.

Down the unlit hall.

Stood in front of the door to the lobby.

Open the door.

I couldn't.

But I couldn't go back to the dressing room to face Viva, either.

OPEN IT.

I watched my hand reach out. I grasped the doorknob, and turned it. I opened the door.

There was a man in the lobby, standing in front of the desk. He seemed relaxed. He didn't seem visibly appalled by the smell of the lobby, or the ambient filth, or the weird network of cords criss-crossing the lobby to power the buzzing neon sign and the broken fluorescent panel. As I stepped through the doorway, he looked me up and down and smiled.

"You new?" he said.

"Yeah," I said. I stared at the carpet.

There was a long silence. Finally, he said, "Uh, I'm here for a session."

I said, "Sixty dollars. Sir. But I can get the other girl. She's totally pretty. I completely understand. Let me just—"

"Nah, that's okay," he said. "You'll do fine."

You'll do fine. Continuing to stare at the carpet, I stepped backward through the doorway. "Follow me," I said.

"Don't you want the money first?" the customer asked. It occurred to me that he was laughing at me. He sounded—*merry,* I guess. Humored.

I put my hand out. He handed me three twenty-dollar bills. They were crisp and new.

I crumpled them into a ball and held them in one fist. I turned and walked down the hall. He followed.

"Can I use the restroom first?" he asked. I pointed down the hall to the bathroom. He went in. I heard running water. Then silence. Then more running water. Then he came out, drying his hands on a paper towel, which he turned and tossed back into the garbage can inside the door.

"We're in here, sir," I said, pointing toward the larger of the two veal pens—the one Crystal and I had used. The customer entered the room, and I shut the door behind him.

I walked back into the lounge. Took off my stupid Payless shoes. Shoved them in my backpack. Took off my tank top, and the horrible humiliating too-small skirt. I was never, ever, ever going to wear any of this, ever again. I was going to burn everything. There was no fucking way. *No fucking way.*

"Did you get his money?" Viva leaned in the doorway. She'd drawn in eyebrows, two thin, brown arcs above her eyes, like a Roaring Twenties flapper.

"Yeah," I said. I opened my fist and showed her the limp bills, all wet and sad from the sweat of my palm. I let them fall to the floor. "But no. There's no way. I am not doing this."

"Yeah, you are," Viva said.

"You want the money? Here. Take it. I don't care. I'm not going in there."

"Yeah," she repeated, "you are." She turned and walked out of the lounge.

I imagined knocking on the door and handing the money back to the customer. Then I imagined simply pushing the bills under the door, on my way out.

I couldn't think of how to escape.

What's the worst that could happen? I thought. I had no answer to that. *You only have to do this once,* I thought. *Then you can leave and never come back, ever again.*

I put my Payless shoes back on and pulled the men's suit jacket out of my backpack. I shook the coat out and put it on, leaving the twenties on the floor next to the couch where I'd dropped them.

I went down the stairs and into the hall and rapped on the door of the veal pen, hard, like a cop. I didn't wait for an answer—I just opened the door and stepped in. I was on autopilot. The man was naked, sitting on the same towel I'd sat on while I watched Crystal do her show. I saw skin, hairy legs, bare feet. His thighs were spread apart. He wasn't looking at the magazines. He had just been waiting. I noticed he'd moved the baby oil. It was closer to the couch—more convenient. The top of the bottle was flipped open. I kept my eyes down, walked over to the boom box, and pressed Play.

Then I stood up. And I started to dance.

I wore the suit jacket for a while, opening and closing it the way I thought a stripper would—teasing the customer with flashes of skin and lingerie. In retrospect, I probably looked like a child-molesting flasher. I noticed my customer's hand pistoning in his lap, but I couldn't see his cock. That was a relief.

Eventually I dropped the coat on the floor and kicked it over next to the boom box.

By the second song, I stood there in my Payless shoes, my ripped stockings, my bra, and my thong. I was breathing hard from moving around—dancing quickly, the way I'd do at a club. My back was sweaty.

I had been keeping my front toward the customer, and my butt turned away from him. I didn't want him to see my fat, jiggly ass and demand his money back. But by the middle of the second song, I was out of things to do, and winded from dancing so hard. So I turned around.

He moaned.

I spun back around. Stared at him. Was he making fun of me?

"You have a beautiful ass," the customer said. His hand kept going up and down. The smell of baby oil, heated by skin friction, filled the room. "Spread those cheeks for me."

I turned around and did as he asked. The whole thing was unreal. The music was too loud. If he attacked me, would anyone help me? Would Viva rescue me? What if he tried to shoot his cum on me? Was it okay to spread myself open like this? I didn't remember Crystal doing anything like that. I felt like livestock—a big fat cow, with some farmer's hand up my snatch. I held my ass cheeks apart and waited.

He moaned and shifted on the couch. When I turned back to check on him, he was wiping his hands on a washcloth.

"Are you done?" I asked him.

"Yeah," he said.

"Okay," I said. I grabbed my coat, put it on, and walked out of the room. I stood in the hall outside the veal pen, trembling. Was I going to get fired for what I just did? The spreading? Were they allowed to ask for that?

A few minutes later, the customer opened the door and came out, fully dressed. I walked him down the dark hall in silence, opening the lobby door for him.

"Thank you," he said. He left. *Beeeeeeeep.*

I went back to the veal pen and looked on the table. There was another crisp twenty-dollar bill on top of one of the magazines, next to the wadded-up washcloth he'd used to clean his hands.

A tip.

Mine.

I'd just made $40.

When I was working as a barista, serving coffee and giving people their change, I'd been making $5 an hour. Before taxes. I worked fifty-five hours a week, plus all the extra shifts I could get, and I still couldn't afford to go to a matinee or order a pizza or buy a pair of shoes that weren't cracked and stinking and secondhand.

But here—just now, in ten minutes—I'd made the equivalent of eight hard, humiliating hours of work. Eight hours on my feet, getting screamed at by customers and managers and whoever else needed to take out their rage on someone who had absolutely no power, who couldn't say anything back, who needed the money desperately enough to put up with the abuse and constant exhaustion.

Ten minutes. Forty dollars.

I began to cry.

I cried all the way back to the lounge, where I picked up the rest of my money. I held it in my hands, protecting it.

Viva came in, looked at me on the floor, and walked back out without comment.

"Celebrity" — Bile

I ended up making $90 on my first shift as a Live Lingerie Adult Model. I came back on Friday morning for my next shift and made $60. I came back on Saturday morning, worked a double shift, and made over $200. I was in love with Butterscotch's. I was even getting used to the smell. I'd also figured a few things out.

One of the first things I did, on a tip from Crystal after my second shift, was go to Broadway Boutique and buy two evening dresses. One was black with silver spangles, the other red stretch velvet. Neither of them cost more than $19. Both of them were tiny, cut for the child-size Asian women who worked and shopped there. I poured myself into those dresses and was pleased at how they made my bust and hips look so big, and my waist look so little. Crystal called them my Jessica Rabbit dresses, since they made me look as much like the freakishly hourglass-shaped übervixen in *Who Framed Roger Rabbit?* as a human could. She was also pleased with me for painting my fingernails and toenails bright, matching red. The polish had gotten all over my hands, but it came off after I soaked my hands in warm water and scrubbed the stained skin with a nailbrush.

I bought long, satin gloves at Broadway Boutique, as well. They were only $15. They made me feel like an Old West saloon girl. I experimented with wearing them throughout my lingerie show. I looked in the smoked glass mirror and saw a girl in tarty black satin underwear and long, shiny black gloves, and I liked what I saw.

I learned to control every part of my costume that I took off—to place it far away from the customer, and to take everything with me whenever I left the room. I learned that customers would steal anything from their "fantasy girl," given the chance. Money carelessly left on the table could be snatched back by a stingy client after his orgasm, the bills having served their temporary purpose as a way to elicit a hotter show—so I learned to seize tips immediately, and to tuck them into my bra or stocking.

I went to Walgreens and bought makeup. Lots of makeup. Eye shadow, eyeliner, foundation, powder, even blush. I paid close attention when Viva put hers on, and I tried to copy her the best I could. I still couldn't put on the liquid eyeliner right, but I loved my red Wet 'n' Wild lipstick and wore it every day I worked.

I replaced the men's suit jacket with a lacy slip that I bought at Target on sale for $5.99. The lace felt scratchy, but it looked feminine and pretty. The customers loved that lace slip. Some of them even asked me to keep it on throughout their sessions. I learned to pull the straps of the slip off my shoulders, and pull the skirt up in little teasing flashes. *Now you see panties, now you don't.* I felt like Marilyn Monroe standing on the subway grate in *The Seven Year Itch,* flipping my skirt around innocently like I didn't even know the tops of my stockings and the front part of my panties were showing. I wasn't sure why occasional glimpses of panty were better than an unobstructed, complete view, but it seemed like the less I showed, the more excited the customers got. I realized they liked to beg for more and be denied.

I got used to turning around, facing the wall, and arching my back, hard. I'd always thought my ass was too big. I didn't realize that the kind of men who liked women's asses tended to adore big, round, jiggly butts, just like mine. I got kind of vain about my bottom, and got lazy in my routine. Sometimes I'd just walk into the session, turn around, arch my back, and shake my ass until the customer had his orgasm. That way I didn't have to look into their faces or endure them staring into mine.

I learned to watch them in the mirrors while I was turned around, so if they leapt up to touch me I could put the metal dancer chair between us, blocking their way. I handled that kind of misbehavior by telling them, "Sit down! *Now!*" firmly, the way you instruct dogs.

I shaved my body every other day. It seemed like half of my life was spent in the bathtub, running a pink razor over my crotch and legs. Crystal told me to put deodorant on my crotch after shaving to keep red razor bumps from forming. It stung, but it worked.

I started looking at the customers' cocks, amazed at the variety that existed. Some were very small, comparable to the size of my thumb. Some were enormous. Most of them stank, in varying degrees. The dense and fungal aromas emanating from the customers' private parts reminded me of cheese, urine, and old butter.

Their assholes frequently smelled of shit. More often than not I'd pick up the bath towel after a session only to find a brown stripe of smeared feces dead center, where my customer had been sitting. I wondered how it felt to walk around with an unwiped asshole, and how their wives felt about doing their shit-streaked laundry. I figured that most men didn't care if their bodies were disgusting because they could pay women like me to pretend not to notice their lack of hygiene. I joked to Heather that seventy-five cents on the dollar meant that men could smell of shit, and women couldn't.

I started bringing latex gloves to pick up the towels after the sessions.

I figured out that most of the smell of Butterscotch's was men's bodies, and their ejaculatory fluid. The rest of it was the chemicals we used to cover up the rich stink of our customers.

A few weeks after my first shift at Butterscotch's, I heard from Heather that Lenore was coming back from L.A.

A day later, I was in the dressing room putting on makeup. The front door went *beep beep beeeeeeeep,* and a moment later Lenore appeared.

I was shocked.

In her flat-soled Doc Martens boots, she was shorter than I remembered her. With no makeup on, her skin was battered with old acne scars and freckles. Marks from obsolete piercings made tiny dents near her eyebrows and mouth. She was still pretty, but she looked so *hard.* And her long, silky black hair—it was gone. Instead, her hair was brown, and ratted into messy dreadlocks. Her shoulders looked broad, out of proportion with her narrow hips and her short legs.

She tossed her backpack onto the counter. "Hey," she said. "Emma, right? Viva said you got hired." She pulled her patched sweatshirt off, revealing a Neurosis shirt and armfuls of blurry tattoos.

This was Lenore? Where was Bettie Page? Where was the girl in the blue velvet dress, so gracious and confident and elegant? Who was this gutter punk?

"You did your hair . . . ?" I asked. "In L.A. . . . ?"

"My hair?" Suddenly Lenore laughed. "Oh my god, no. Are you serious? I wear a wig here. Customers hate punk rock girls."

A wig. I'd had no idea.

Lenore undressed. I noticed she was wearing thong panties under her jeans.

"Do you like it here?" she asked, squinting at me. "You seriously didn't know that was a wig? God, I feel like everyone knows, as soon as they walk in the door. It's like freakin' doll hair."

"Yeah," I said. "And no, I didn't."

"That's hilarious," she said.

I wasn't sure what to make of this new Lenore. In some ways I liked her better: She was less intimidating, more like a girl I'd hang out with in real life. But her coolness opened up its own set of problems. Girls like Lenore scared the shit out of me, made me shy and speechless. I didn't know how to talk to someone who was that punk rock.

"How was L.A.?" I asked.

"Fine. I hung out with my mom, and did some shit, and got some of my stuff out of storage. It's good to be back, though. My dogs missed me." Lenore was putting on makeup: first concealer, then foundation, then pressed powder. Magically, her skin looked flawless again. It was like an optical illusion. I had to remind myself that underneath her makeup there were dents and scars and blotches. It was amazing.

I wanted that. I wanted to transform.

She opened her pack and pulled out a plastic bag. Her wig. She took it out of the bag and brushed it briskly. It looked like a shiny black pet.

After her hairpiece was smooth and untangled, she pinned it on carefully, using the combs inside the fibrous netted cap to attach it at her hairline. Then she took out a bottle of liquid eyeliner, raised her chin, and made her eyes into slits. In two smooth motions, she drew lines right above her eyelashes, winging the outer edges up in swoops. I was breathless. It looked so pretty.

"That's so cool," I said. "I love the way you do your eye makeup."

"Want me to put some on you?"

I couldn't believe it. "Yeah," I said.

"Tilt your head up. Now kind of close your eyes," she said. The tiny brush felt cold against my eyelid. "Don't fucking blink!"

I didn't blink. My eyes started watering.

"Now I'm gonna do the other side," she said. It felt like she was drawing the line all the way over to my temple. As the liquid eyeliner dried, it tightened on my skin.

"Lenore?"

"Huh?"

"Can I blink now?"

"Oh! Yeah, go ahead," she said. "It looks nice."

I looked in the mirror. I couldn't believe how good I looked. I looked like a model. I was perfect. I couldn't take my eyes off my lips, full and red, and my eyes, so dark and tilted up at the corners, thanks to the liquid liner. I wanted to stay that way forever. A little voice in my head whispered, *You're prettier than Lenore.*

Beeep beeeep beeeeeeeeeeeeeep. It sounded like a stupid customer standing right in the door buzzer's light sensor. *Beeeeeeeeeeeep.*

"Move *forward,* dick!" said Lenore. She looked at me. "You're up."

"I know," I said. I put on my gloves and clumped down the stairs and through the hall to the front door.

The guy standing in the lobby was small and hip looking. He had a leather coat on, cut '70s-style, but not like he bought it secondhand. It was like it was cut *ironically,* like it was super expensive but made to look like some pimp coat from Goodwill, just to make fun of people who couldn't afford to buy fancy leather coats.

"Hi," I said. "Have you been here before?"

"No," the hipster said. He looked around, sniffing the horrible, musty air and looking concerned. I tried to play it off like I couldn't smell anything. I sat in the broken desk chair, lounging elegantly. I'd learned that louche, mannered sprawl from watching all the other girls while they talked to their customers.

I went into the spiel I'd learned from Heather on my second day at Butterscotch's. "What we offer is a *very sexy* live lingerie show. You go into a private room with your own model. She'll go down to a *very sexy* bra and thong panty. You can get as comfortable as you like during your session"—code for *You can spank it like a spider monkey*—"as long as there's no touching between yourself and your model. Remember, you can enjoy yourself completely"—

blow your load into a washcloth—"and then after your session, your tan is complimentary. Would you like to try a session?"

"Uh," he said. "Who's my model?"

"The girl who greets you at the door is usually your model for your session," I said. "I'm Emma."

We stared at each other.

"Uh, okay," he said. "Is that like Emma Peel?"

"Would you like a fantasy session?" I asked him. "That's where I can talk dirty to you, and explore your wildest fantasies."

We stared at each other again.

"Um, sure," he said. "Is that extra?"

"It's eighty dollars," I said. "The dirty talk is only twenty dollars more than the regular. But it's a much, much hotter show."

"I don't know," he said.

"It's our sexiest show," I said. "If you've never tried anything like this before, it'll probably blow your mind."

He took out his money—a hundred-dollar bill.

"Thanks, honey," I said. I tucked the bill into my bra. I didn't offer change, and he didn't mention it. *Sucker.*

As I walked the hipster down the hall, I added it up. Eighty dollars minus forty to the house, plus twenty extra, meant sixty dollars for me.

I felt like singing.

After I put him in our veal pen, I went back to the dressing room. Lenore was wearing the blue dress I remembered from the first time I saw her. She still seemed short without her shoes on—her legs seemed about the length of my arms. Having seen the *real* Lenore, the dressed-up Lenore was somehow less compelling. Or maybe it was that I couldn't stop staring past her into the mirror. My eyes looked huge with all that black makeup on.

"Didja get him?" she said.

"Yeah."

"Cool."

I spritzed myself with vanilla body spray and took off my black and silver evening gown. I put on my lacy slip and adjusted my stockings so they were nice and neat, and weren't rolling down at the top. The heat was up high, and it felt good. It made my muscles feel loose and warm. I'd made sixty bucks, and the shift was only just getting started. I felt like it was going to be a really good day.

"Okay," I said.

"Have an erotic time," said Lenore.

"Ha ha," I said. "I can't wait to really *connect* with this guy, *emotionally.*" I was still nervous walking into the showroom, even though I'd done a bunch of shows already. It was nerve-racking. You never knew what your customer was going to be like. As ridiculous as it was to strip down to a bra and thong and walk around grabbing your own breasts and ass, you could always get a guy who would try to touch you, or who would try to demand more nudity. It happened. You had to be careful. Joking around with the other girls made it a little easier. "We *connect* through the sacred gift of *sensuality.*"

Lenore put her lipstick down and laughed.

I stepped into the hall and opened the door to my veal pen.

The hipster was sitting there in the dark, on his towel, nude. He had leather cuffs around his wrists. Next to him on the towel were two metal cock rings and his own personal container of lube. It was open.

"I thought you didn't know what we did here," I said.

"I called a few days ago," he said. "I talked to a girl on the phone. She kind of told me how it works."

"So why'd you make me go through the spiel, dreamboat?" I asked. I liked calling customers *dreamboat, dollface, lover, sugar pie.* All those dumb terms of pseudoendearment. I felt like a gangster's moll, saying them. Besides, I could never remember to ask them their names.

"Did you just like the pretty sound of my voice, buttercup?" I laughed. I had been working on my laugh. It was softer, more giggly, less loud and brash. I was pretty happy with it. It wasn't a purr like Lenore's—yet. But it was still more like clinking ice cubes in a tall, cool glass of gin than I ever thought I could sound. I found that laughing at customers disarmed them; it made them tentative, like big, shy boys. I laughed when I needed time to think, or when I wasn't sure what to say.

I was learning so much.

"I wanted to make sure it was still the same thing," he said. His cock lurched, stirring against his thigh. It was surprisingly big for such a small guy, and curved, like a fat sausage. I towered over him.

"Let's get started, sexy," I said. I turned on my CD but kept the volume low. I'd brought a mix of Beck songs culled from his first couple of albums—the slower, more acoustic ones. I liked Beck Hansen's weary growl and definitive, quirky percussion much better than the electronica some girls used, which seemed too fast and sterile. I wanted the veal pen—as smelly and filthy as it was—to at least *sound* like a bedroom, not a club. All that techno beeping and hooting, and those embarrassing drum machines—I didn't see how we were supposed to create a mood with that. Even worse was R&B. I'd heard a few girls doing shows to that. *Baby baby, let me do it to you all night*—I couldn't imagine how the customers stayed hard with that playing.

Viva used a weird, scary mix of industrial and metal, but Viva could do whatever she wanted to do and the customers would still come back and see her again and again. I didn't know what she did in her shows. She was so imperious, so surly and strange. I couldn't imagine her even smiling at the customers, let alone allowing them to masturbate while looking at her. But they loved her. She was one of the most requested models at Butterscotch's.

I stood up, making eye contact with the hipster. I looked at him and thought, *I want to fuck you so bad.* I thought, *Get your cock*

hard and fuck me. Now. I found when I thought things like that—
even if they weren't true—the customers got aroused much faster.

I'd learned not to dance in my sessions—dancing was amateur.
I remembered how Crystal had showed me all her lovely parts, over
and over, in different ways, and how slow and fluid her motions
were. I tried to show the customers all my parts, slowly, giving
them time to really look. That and eye contact. It was actually
pretty easy.

"So, what are you into?" I asked. "You have any particular
fantasies . . . ?"

"Yeah," the hipster said. His shoulders were so narrow. "I
love your ass."

"Oh yeah?" I said. Autopilot. "Well, I want you to bend me
over this chair and spank my nice, big, round ass."

"Yeah?" He started rubbing his cock.

"Uh-huh," I said. "I've got a few other things I'd like you to
do to my big, luscious ass, too. Wanna hear about them?"

We were off.

Ten minutes later, I handed him a clean washcloth, watched
him dress, and walked him to the front door.

This was absolutely the best job I'd ever had.

After three months at Butterscotch's, I threw my old white cotton
bikini panties away. They didn't feel good anymore. They felt like
bloomers, or those freaky Mormon underwear singlets, or diapers.
Now I proudly bought my panties out of bins, not in old-lady
packages. The different colors in my underwear drawer looked
sexy and intoxicating. Every morning I'd pick which ones to wear,
and all day long I'd think, *I'm wearing the red lace pair,* or *I'm
wearing the black see-through ones with the pink bows.* It made
me feel like anything could happen.

For the first time in my life, I had begun to feel more desirable than not. It was like winning the lottery, or losing my mind—my approach to everything became different. Once you make the assumption that everyone thinks you're beautiful, the world becomes a strange and lovely place. And the more beautiful you think you are, the more the world treats you that way. I got used to people complimenting me, trying to talk to me, giving me things, letting me go first. Beautiful girls get all kinds of treats. I loved them all, couldn't get enough of them. I'd never had those treats before.

I got thinner.

I plucked my eyebrows out until they were just skinny lines, like the ones Viva drew on before every shift.

I realized I had a real facility for this kind of work—"adult" work. It agreed with me. I could say *Fuck my ass* and *I'm gonna fucking come* and *I wanna suck your cock* with a straight face. I could make those phrases fresh and believable. Every time I said something filthy, I expected a customer to say *All right, now that's just ridiculous,* but that never happened. My customers' capacity for suspension of belief was without boundary.

My sessions became Grand Guignol. My words were surreal and sickening, like a page from the Marquis de Sade with priests fucking nuns and virgins getting deflowered by their own fathers and daisy chains of people screwing each other and being screwed in various inventive and scatological permutations. My dirty talk was so full of corruption that even when I said, *Oh, kiss me, sweet baby,* my intonation turned it into something macabre and grossly perverse. My fantasy shows weren't even erotic. They were Krafft-Ebing, not Nancy Friday. They were freak shows.

And along with Viva, I became one of the more asked-for models.

Chapter 2
Real Live Horny Girl Next Door

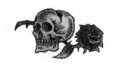

"Bitches" —
Mindless Self Indulgence

Every Thursday the local alternative paper *The Stranger* came out, and every Friday morning I went to Cafe Roma to pick up a free copy. Later, once I was in costume and waiting for customers at Butterscotch's, I'd look under Adult Help Wanted for modeling jobs. Adult Help was a subset of the regular Help Wanted section, with calls for local escorts, dancers, and nude models. Until I'd started working at Butterscotch's, I'd never even noticed that section of the classified ads before. The text was surrounded by big ads for phone sex, pornographic websites, and the services of local prostitutes. The saddest escort ads were the ones with bleary camera-phone pictures next to the pager numbers.

Crystal had inspired me to look through the Adult Help Wanted ads for photo and web modeling work to supplement my wages as a live lingerie model. She modeled constantly when she wasn't at Butterscotch's—she had a portfolio and her own website. She'd shown me some of her pictures, and I was astonished at how different she looked in photographs: taller, with bright makeup that transformed her tired skin into glowing ivory. In her pictures, Crystal looked strong, confident, and glamorous.

She did a lot of shoots for local bondage aficionados, so most of her pictures showed her tied up or bound in some way, with a ball gag in her mouth. In some of the pictures she was the dominant, and in those she posed with leather paddles or gestured to her scarily

high-heeled shoes. Her expressions didn't change much, regardless
of whether she was bound with rope or brandishing a snaky, coiled
bullwhip: Whatever her predicament, her face was stony and calm.
Her dispassion was strangely sexy. It was like she didn't know or
didn't care about what was happening to her; like she was so absent
that you could fantasize whatever you wanted about her, no matter
how filthy, and none of it would matter. She did some standard
"adult work" as well, but nothing with her legs spread, she said.

Privately, I figured that if Crystal could model, so could I.

Plus, I was willing to spread my legs.

I let Crystal know that if any of her photographers needed a
tall, curvy brunette, I wanted to work. And every week I read Adult
Help Wanted, looking for ads that didn't seem creepy—or that at
least didn't sound dangerous. I called some of them, but if the men
answering the phone sounded like they were touching themselves
while talking to me—or if they tried to pressure me to come to
their studios immediately, or if they didn't even have studios and
just worked out of their own homes—I made excuses and hung
up. One photographer was so angry with me for calling him, and
then not agreeing to model for him, that he reverse-dialed me and
screamed, "Whore! Lying whore!" into the phone, then slammed
it down. After that happened, I became even more cautious.

One ad in particular attracted me. It said:

*Are you plump, with an hourglass figure? Nationally known
photographer seeks models of all shapes, sizes, and weights. Be an
XXX star! No experience necessary!*

I watched the ad run for several weeks in a row. I figured that
meant it was at least a little bit legitimate. I mean, if the guy were
inviting models to his studio, and then chopping their heads off
or raping them, wouldn't the Seattle Police Department make *The
Stranger* pull his ads?

I dialed the number.

"Yes?" There was noise in the background—it sounded like his TV was on.

"Hi," I said. "I'm calling about your ad? In *The Stranger?*"

"Yeah . . . hang on." The TV sounds abruptly ended. "Which one?"

"Um . . . 'Are you plump, with an hourglass figure?'"

"Oh yeah. So, *are* you?"

I hated this part. Every photographer I called wanted me to describe myself, and every time I paused and had no idea what to say. I was never sure how detailed to get.

"I'm curvy," I said. "I have blue eyes. Shoulder-length brown hair."

"Do you have any tattoos or piercings?"

"I have a few tattoos," I said. "My navel's pierced. Is that a problem?"

"No," the photographer said. "Not necessarily. How old are you?"

"Twenty," I said. I could pass for twenty, though I was really twenty-four. I'd learned to lie about my age at Butterscotch's. We all did it. Customers liked to think they were getting someone young and fresh.

It was weird: They went to a place like Butterscotch's, as dank as it was, and they expected to find their girl-next-door Dulcinea amid the filth. But if we really *were* that innocent, why would we be working in a place where we made money by watching men masturbate to us? The kind of girls they really wanted were all working as daycare teachers, professional cheerleaders, librarians, or nurses—or they were in college studying something midrange and practical, like marketing or communications. Expecting to find a sweet, sincere, corn-fed coed in a place like Butterscotch's was utter insanity. But they all tried. They loved to think we were only in Butterscotch's by some kind of weird mistake.

I'd had countless customers tell me, "You don't belong here. You're too beautiful to be here. You're too innocent—too sweet!"

Of course, they tended to say this as they were pounding away at themselves, sitting on a bath towel, with baby-oiled fingers shoved deep inside their own rectums.

I'd just giggle, spread my legs, and marvel at the massive cognitive dissonance necessary for men to believe that the women they'd paid to perform sexual acts were actually *doing* those sexual acts of their own volition instead of for the money. The whole virgin/whore question wasn't about which one they wanted—the secret was they wanted *both,* at the same time, in the same girl. That was their "fantasy girl"—a female they could pay $60 to jerk off to, and then take home to Mom.

In a weird way, though, we *were* all nice, decent girls. We were kind to each other: We covered each other's shifts and brought each other cake and presents on birthdays. But we also spread our ass cheeks, got on our hands and knees, and pretended to masturbate—for money, in front of strangers. All I knew is that it seemed like every man wanted to be our first. Every customer wanted to pretend that his cock was the only one we'd ever seen. But at the same time, they had to know that if we'd take their money, we'd take anyone's.

"Twenty, huh?" said the photographer. He sounded like a New York Jew, surprisingly. I was a little charmed in spite of myself.

"I'm a girl-next-door type," I said. In industry terminology, that meant I was white with decent teeth—not too glamorous or vampy, and not overly tattooed or made up. The opposite of "girl next door" was "sophisticated," or "exotic." *Sophisticated* meant old, and *exotic* meant nonwhite. If you were sophisticated *and* exotic, you were a niche market, at best.

"Let me tell you a little bit about myself," said the photographer. I heard him switch the phone from one ear to the other.

"You may have heard of me—my name is Roderick Saxon. I'm an award-winning adult filmmaker, based here in Seattle, and also L.A. I specialize in first-person amateur stuff—where the guys watching can feel like they're right in there with the beautiful girls themselves. I've been making films and videos for fifteen years."

I could tell that he was a little disappointed that I didn't recognize his name.

"Have you heard of 'Buttman'? John Stagliano?"

"Uh, no," I said. I felt bad. "I'm sorry. I, uh, don't rent a lot of adult videos."

We sat in silence.

"You *do* know what this ad is for, don't you?" Roderick asked suddenly.

"Modeling? Nude?"

"Yeah," he said. "And maybe some video work, if you look good and I like working with you."

I didn't know why—maybe it was his yeshiva school accent—but I wanted to work for Roderick. He wasn't masturbating to me on the phone, trying to breathe heavily away from the receiver as he talked to me. He sounded professional. And he actually seemed *wounded* that I hadn't recognized his name, which made me feel protective of him. He'd exuded pride when he'd said *Let me tell you a little about myself,* like he was going to say who he was and I was supposed to squeal and clap my hands and go *Oh my god, it's you! I can't believe it!* And here I was not even knowing his name, or even John Stagliano from "Buttman," whatever that was. I wondered if he and "Buttman" were partners.

"When are you free? Can you come in, let's see . . ." I heard pages flipping. It reassured me. Most of the creeps posting fake model calls in *The Stranger* didn't have appointment books. They just tried to get you to come to their "studios" immediately.

"How's tomorrow afternoon?"

I had to work the day shift at Butterscotch's. "Uh, can we make it the day after? That's my next day off."

"Oh? Where do you work?"

I told him.

"Oh!" He sounded pleased. "Great! Yeah, definitely the next day, that's fine. Bring photo ID, and be ready to work. You have costumes, I take it?"

I did. "Do you want anything in particular . . . Roderick?" I'd learned to ask clients that. If they wanted me to put on something special—the most usual requests were stockings and a garter belt—I charged them $20 extra. I wasn't planning on charging Roderick; the question was just automatic. Plus, that way I wouldn't have to pack everything and end up not using a bunch of stuff he didn't like.

"No, no," he said. "Just look like a sexy, normal girl. But don't look too strippery—remember, this is amateur. They want girls that look like real girls, not pros. The guys buying this want to feel like they could really have a chance with you. Get it?"

I certainly did. In other words, he was looking for what every customer at Butterscotch's seemed to want: a nice, normal, sweet girl who would strip down to whorish underwear and get nasty for cash.

"Somewhat Damaged"— Nine Inch Nails

I showed up at Roderick's condo right on time and buzzed his number, as directed. The security system asked me for the pass code, and I keyed it in: 6969. It figured.

I rode the elevator up. His building was one of those brand-new, horrible "luxury" condos that littered Capitol Hill, cracker boxes with thin walls and exorbitant maintenance fees that had rapidly replaced most of the beautiful old brick buildings where working-class folks and artists used to live. Everything in Roderick's building looked cheap and terrible, from the manufactured "paintings" on the walls to the shoddy beige carpeting underfoot. Living there would be like living in a Ramada Inn. His building looked like a hotel, smelled like a hotel, and yet was somehow less gracious than a hotel. I bet he didn't even have an ice machine.

Yet, I guessed from the location, his condo probably cost more than half a million dollars. I couldn't believe the things that people spent their money on. But then again, he was from L.A., wasn't he? Maybe he didn't know how ugly and depressing the new luxury condos were. Or maybe he thought that's how people lived here.

The elevator doors opened silently. I stepped out, shouldering my backpack, which was crammed full of "nice, normal girl" costumes. There were some men painting the hallway, so I had to pick my way over the plastic drop cloth on the floor on my way to Roderick's door. The workmen stared at me. I knew they knew I didn't live there. I knocked, and a very tall, very thin man opened the door. "Hi," he said. "Pleased to meet you. Come on in." He stepped back, and I entered his apartment. It was him—I knew him by his voice right away: the New York Jewish pornographer from L.A. *Roderick Saxon.*

He wore a splashy Hawaiian shirt, unbuttoned down to his sternum. Dark hair showed in the V of his collar, but thankfully, no gold medallion was visible. He wore wire-framed glasses with bright pink-tinted lenses. The tinting made his eyes look muddy and expressionless. His nose was valiantly beaky. Between that and the shirt, he looked like a parrot.

His hair was frizzy and pubic, cut long in the back and on top, and shorter on the sides. A Jewish afro-mullet. It was medium brown with a few threads of gray snarled through.

This is the famous pornographer? I thought.

"Well, look at you," Roderick said. "Heidi, right?"

"Uh-huh," I said. I was sick of being Emma. Too many customers had wrecked that name for me, and now when I heard it, I cringed. I didn't think of Emma Goldman when I heard it anymore. All I could think of was men moaning and thrashing on their towels, squeezing their cocks into their hands, then slurping up their own ejaculate or wiping it onto the exposed fabric of the couch.

I had chosen the name Heidi from Johanna Spyri's novel about Heidi of the Alps, the adorable moppety goat girl. I'd liked that book a lot when I was little; I'd wanted a dress with an embroidered panel on the front and a white apron, and most of all I'd wanted to drink fresh, warm goat's milk out of a wooden bowl.

It sounded so sweet and good. That was my favorite part of the book, when Heidi drank the goat's milk.

I also thought *Heidi* suited me. I tended to wear my hair in two braids, parted in the middle, and I was fair and sturdy and blue-eyed, like a German *Mädchen* or a Hummel figurine. It seemed like the name might excite the same kind of men who thought the St. Pauli *bier* girl was hot. Plus there was an aspect of sexual tourism I'd noticed at Butterscotch's: The customers really liked "types"—the Asian pearl of the Orient, or the red-haired Irish lassie, or the fiery, dark-complected Latina. If you could play it off like you were a certain purebred something, it didn't seem to matter what that something was. The customers would take at least one show with you, as if they were checking items off a list on a scavenger hunt. Faking a convincing accent could be incredibly profitable.

I think it was kind of like that old saying about "a girl in every port"—but men who couldn't afford to travel could at least pay $60 to jack off to the kind of girl they'd never meet in real life. Going to a place like Butterscotch's reinforced their fantasy of themselves as sexual adventurers. It was like the Westminster Kennel Club Dog Show, but with girls instead of dogs: Every man wanted to frolic with the best of each breed, the fancy, expensive, temperamental purebreds—even if he had a certain affection for his own life companion, the faithful mutt left in the kennel at home.

So I was Heidi—long-legged, busty, fair, and utterly Aryan. Standing in front of Roderick for inspection, it occurred to me that we looked like something out of a Woody Allen film: the ultimate Jew, and the ultimate shiksa.

"Look at *you*," he said again.

I smiled. I tucked my cheeks back to make dimples, the way I'd learned to do.

I noticed Roderick's hands were very big, with long fingers. I wondered if his mother had forced him to take piano lessons as a boy.

Roderick arranged the lights while I went to his anonymous little hotel-room-size bathroom to change into my first costume. As directed, I wanted to look *real*: like a sweet kindergarten teacher who'd just happened to stumble into a pornographer's den, and then stayed to pose for a few pictures.

I dressed in white cotton panties and a matching lacy full-coverage bra. I rolled white thigh-high stockings up my legs, and buckled chunky white high-heeled sandals on my feet. I'd left all my stiletto-heeled shoes at home, rejecting them as too strippery. Over my lingerie, I wore a black-and-white-checked gingham sundress, sleeveless, with a sash that tied in the back to shape it through the waist. Except for the fact that the skirt on the dress was mid-thigh length, I looked like I was ready to go to Mass.

I unbraided my hair and clipped it back with little white flowered barrettes.

My makeup was simple: powder, to make my skin tone appear more even. Deep pink lipstick. Mascara.

I came out of the bathroom. Roderick was still moving lights around. A big sheet of fabric hung as a backdrop behind a small, low-backed couch, which had been pulled away from the wall to allow photographic angles from all sides. Gauzy, multicolored scarves had been draped randomly over the couch. It was already hot from the big clamp lights, and Roderick sweated as he adjusted them. I could see the pores on his nose from where I stood.

"Is this okay?" I asked. I spread my arms out at my sides.

"Turn around," Roderick said. I turned slowly, then back again, to face him.

"I don't know if you're chubby enough for this series," he said. "It's called *Fat, Horny Bitches 3*. And you're not fat."

"Yeah, I am," I said. "I'm thick. I've got big thighs, and a big butt."

"I don't know," he said. He seemed disappointed. "Maybe you could be in my regular series, *Here's Cum in Your Eye.* We're up to number eight on that title."

I couldn't believe we were arguing about how fat I was. All my life I'd been yelled at and made fun of for being too big. When I walked into Butterscotch's, I was terrified that they wouldn't even want to give me an application because I weighed over 150 pounds. Now I was trying to convince a pornographer that I was overweight enough to be in a photo shoot for something called *Fat, Horny Bitches 3.*

"Please, Roderick," I said. "I want to be in *Fat, Horny Bitches.* Not *Here's Cum in Your Eye.* The guys who like chubby girls will like me, I promise. I'm fatter looking with my clothes off." I'd taken the day off work and taken the bus all the way to his condo. I didn't want to be turned away summarily just because Roderick was scared I wasn't curvy enough to satisfy his hordes of drooling fans. I knew I was—I knew I could do this. Besides, didn't the camera add ten pounds?

"All right, if you feel that strongly about it," he shrugged.

He moved a clamp light so it spotlighted the couch.

"We're going to start with some stills," he said. "Go ahead and get on the couch."

I did. As I put my knees on the couch and arched my back, presenting my ass to Roderick's camera, I thought, *I am making pornography.*

"Okay, look back at me," he said. I did, over one shoulder. I pulled my dress up a little, so the bottom of my panties showed. Suddenly, I smiled.

"Hot," he said.

Click click click.

I am making pornography.

"Holy Diver" — Dio

After about an hour of shooting, I realized that posing for pictures was a lot like doing a show at Butterscotch's—except slower, and with lots of holding still. It was also really, really hot. Even with the big fan Roderick brought in to blow my hair back, the lights made me sweat down my back and between my breasts. I had to keep taking breaks to go into the bathroom to powder the shine off my face. If you didn't do that, you looked greasy, said Roderick.

I'd stripped out of my sundress and out of my bra and was doing some shots where I was pulling my panties up the crack of my ass, as if I were giving myself a wedgie. Once the panties were up my butt crack, I bent over the arm of the couch and spread my legs. Roderick told me to put one hand on each ass cheek, and kind of pull them apart. "Like you're begging for it," he said.

It felt like I spent a lot of time in my life bent over something and pulling my ass cheeks apart. *Probably more than most girls,* I thought.

After more shots, where I finally pulled my panties down to mid-thigh and acted shy, like I didn't know the camera was there—and then slutty, like I did—Roderick called for a break.

I drank bottled water, gulping it down but being careful not to let any of it slosh onto my face. I was so covered in powder that a splash of water would have turned my built-up makeup layers into pancake batter.

"How would you feel about doing a video?" Roderick said. I couldn't see his eyes through his pink-tinted glasses.

"Does it pay more?" I asked.

"Well," he said. "It depends." He paused. "It depends on what we do."

"We?"

"Yeah."

I thought about this for a moment. *We.*

"Uh, Roderick?"

"Yeah?"

"I'm not into getting touched," I said.

"Oh," he said.

"Well," he said. "What if I just kind of, you know, masturbated onto your face?"

"Uh, *no,*" I said. "Actually, for me, that kind of goes under touch."

Roderick looked sad.

"Well, all right," said Roderick, resignedly. I felt like I was twisting his arm.

I finished my water while Roderick went to the closet and pulled down a cardboard box from the upper shelf storage. He brought it over to the couch and opened it up. Inside were about a million dildos, butt plugs, and vibrators, all in similar packaging. Roderick Saxon Presents *Pussy Pounder IX,* said the labels. The packages were decorated with pictures of naked ladies, and a little cartoon of Roderick smoking a cigar. The lenses of his cartoon glasses were pink.

"We had a tie-in with the movie," said Roderick. "These actually sold really well."

They just looked like normal sex toys to me, like anything they'd sell next to blow-up sheep and Fruit Leather panties.

"Uh," I said. "Should I just grab anything?"

"Yeah," he said. "I mean, pick anything that appeals to you."

I rummaged through the box and picked out a medium-size black vibrator. I made sure the box hadn't been opened.

"We also gave these away off the website," Roderick said. "For new subscriptions, and to promote *Pussy Pounder X.*"

I wondered how many Pussy Pounders there ended up being. I mean, ten was a lot.

"Do you want something else?" he asked. He seemed to mean, *Take something else.*

I went through the box again and pulled out a small red dildo in a sealed plastic bag. It was curved, with a flared base, and looked like a pacifier.

"Okay," I said.

It was late afternoon. I felt like I'd been in Roderick's apartment for days. He got up and put the box of toys away, then pulled out a camera tripod and two cameras. One camera went on top of the tripod, which he set up in front of the couch. Then he took batteries out of a black nylon film bag and loaded those into the smaller video camera. "This is the handheld," he said. "They go nuts for handheld. I invented that."

"You invented the *handheld?*"

"No, I mean, using the handheld to film point of view. While I fuck the girl. They like it because it's like they're fucking the girl. They can see everything like they're actually *in* the action. Nobody was doing that before me."

He was proud.

Who would want to watch Roderick Saxon fuck anyone? I thought. He was so gangly, so scrawny, so . . . average. I had assumed male porn stars had to be muscled, tanned, shaved, and conventionally attractive in that Greco-Roman, suspiciously homosexual, manly-man way. Roderick was none of those things. And yet—I thought of *Pussy Pounders X.* I guess if he'd made that many movies, *somebody* had to like watching him fuck. Maybe it was the whole amateur thing of not wanting people to look too good.

"Bathroom," I said. I went in and shut the door.

I took off my panties and used my hands to scoop up warm water from the sink, which I used to wash my pussy. Some of the water dripped down my stockings. I didn't want to use any of his towels, so I dried my puss on the hem of my sundress. Then I used the warm-water-on-the-hands method to clean my asshole. Then I washed my hands with soap, and dried them on my dress. I put my panties back on.

I checked my makeup. It was thick, but fine.

My hair was frizzing a little. Maybe I'd caught the frizz from Roderick. I just hoped I didn't catch anything else from him, from using his toilet or drinking his bottled water or sitting on his gauze-scarf-draped couch.

When I came out of the bathroom, Roderick said we were good to go. He said the larger camera on the tripod was just going to stay on, recording everything from where it was, and that he was going to use the little handheld camera to get in closer and get different angles on the action. From time to time, he said, he was going to ask me to stop moving, so he could grab stills from the images being recorded by the handheld. The stills would be put up on the website to promote the title.

"A lot of the buyers don't have a fast enough Internet connection to look at a ton of little clips from the movies," he explained. "They need stills. For the guys on dial-up, even the stills take a long time to load." He labeled a tape in black Sharpie—*Heidi 1, F. H. Bitches 3,* and the date—and popped it into the handheld.

"Okay," I said. His detached efficiency impressed me. I felt conscious of myself as a product, but the fact that it wasn't personal—that Roderick wasn't primarily motivated by an attraction to me—made me less nervous. Our work together was business: Both of us wanted to get paid. He knew his end of things—the technical stuff—and I knew I could do a good, convincing show. After several months at Butterscotch's, I knew a few tricks.

"You ready?" he asked. I nodded. "Okay, get on the couch, then. I want you to start off with a slow strip. Get real hot, real erotic, like you're getting more and more turned on. Can you talk?"

"Can I . . . ?"

"Talk—can you talk? To the camera?"

"Talk?" I said. "Dirty?"

He nodded.

"Yeah, I think so." I didn't see how that would be any different from talking to a customer.

"Okay, cool. Hang on." He pressed a button on the big camera on the tripod. Nothing changed except a little red light went on right under the lens of the camera. I was being recorded. It made me feel momentarily self-conscious, the way you do when you know you're being watched. I crossed my legs, then uncrossed them. I didn't want to start the video with my legs crossed, looking prissy and uptight.

"Okay, go ahead and start. I'll bring in the handheld in a minute."

I paused. I thought, *Think of this as a live performance. Treat the camera like a customer.*

"Hi," I said. I lowered my voice, tried to get it into my chest and not so much in the mask of my face. I looked into the camera. *It's the customer's eyes,* I thought. *Look into his eyes. Let him know you know he's there.*

"Hi. I'm Heidi. I've been horny all day.

"And now you're watching me, and that makes me even hornier," I said. I ran my hands up my thighs, over my hips, and cupped them under my breasts. Left them there for a moment, as if I were showing them off.

"My nipples are so hard," I said. "Can you see?"

I pulled the hem of my skirt up, exposing the cotton crotch of my panties.

"My pussy's wet. My panties are wet. Can you see?"

Silently, Roderick used the handheld to zoom in on my crotch, then back out again. I spread my legs obligingly.

"Hold," he said. I did. I realized I was holding my breath. It was like playing Freeze Tag.

"Okay, go," he said.

"I want you to fuck me," I said. "But first I want to make your cock nice and hard, so you can fill my pussy up, the way I like it.

"Can I stand?" I asked Roderick, suddenly.

"Yeah, go," said Roderick. "This is good."

I stood, took off my sundress, and sat down again. The couch felt warm under my thighs. The fabric was heated, from the lights. It felt good. The scarves were embarrassing, though, busting Roderick in a transparent attempt at artiness and visual interest.

Roderick was staring at me, the handheld camera strapped to his palm. He frowned a little. *Go,* he mouthed.

"I want you to take my bra off," I said. "I want you to play with my big, round tits. Lick them, suck on them. Squeeze them. You can bite them, a little. That gets me excited."

I unhooked my bra and weighed my breasts in the palms of my hands, like oranges. Handling them was like handling bags of meat. I took the opportunity to check them for lumps, pressing the tissue down with my fingertips as if I were checking to see if a cake was done.

I thought, *It takes doing porn to get me to do a breast self-exam.*

I thought, *I hope I don't find any lumps.*

"I want you to squeeze these big tits together and fuck them. Fuck me," I said. "Shove your cock between them, and make them yours."

Roderick zoomed in on my breasts as I pushed them together.

I moaned. "That feels so good," I said. "Tit-fuck me."

Who liked this?

I wondered if any woman in the world, at any time, any-where, *ever,* had actually achieved orgasm from letting some guy slide his dick in her cleavage. I'd let a boyfriend do it to me, once, but we'd both felt ridiculous.

The astonishing thing about porn is that nobody seems to tire of all the repetition. In every porn movie, varying numbers of dicks, pussies, tits, mouths, and asses get moved around and rearranged and rubbed on each other and shoved into each other. Sometimes there are small, weird variations, but basically, that's *it*—that's porn.

Real sex is far more complicated. Acquiring fluency in sex takes time, like learning a language, and if you do it consistently, maybe at the end of your life you can say that you've mastered it. But not until then. Porn isn't just a poor substitution for the real thing; it's completely unlike real sex in every way. When all you have is body parts, you turn sex into something as reductive and mundane as making a peanut butter and jelly sandwich. I couldn't understand its appeal—wasn't porn's transparent inadequacy insultingly obvious?

I moaned, pressing my tits together and licking my lips. I used my fingertips to pinch my nipples and made sure to arch my back. Body parts.

I thought about my customers at Butterscotch's. They didn't even get to *see* any of those body parts! They paid to just know they were there! It was weird and pathetic—I mean, couldn't you save $60 and just sit next to a pretty girl on the bus, knowing she had a vagina under her pants and panties?

And how come it didn't turn me on to know that men had cocks under their pants? I mean, I knew they had cocks, the same way I knew they had lungs. It didn't excite me. And watching the customers actually take their cocks out and make themselves come—that was just disgusting, like watching a dozen different people blow their noses, one after the other.

I thought of Crystal dancing around in her white thong panties, and about Viva, dressed in her black liquid-looking PVC, her waist cinched in hard by her corset. Were they sexy because they had vaginas under their clothes? Or was it something else?

Ultimately, it was bizarre to me that entire professions rotated around simply *having* vaginas, and *managing* them, as if they were limited environmental resources, like natural gas or diamonds. Roderick's job depended on vagina management: With no vaginas, he'd be completely out of luck and out of business. Butterscotch's ran on vaginas, like trains ran on coal in the old days.

And wasn't I making money hand over fist by deciding when to unveil my own vagina? It seemed like the more you didn't show it, the more people paid you when you finally did.

"It's Tricky" — Run-D.M.C.

I lifted my hips up from the couch and slid my panties off.

"You wanna fingerbang me?" I cooed. "Let's mess around."

I reached down and held my labia open, butterflying my pussy back against my inner thighs. I'd shaved that morning. My skin felt soft. Hair grows back so fast: Less than a day after shaving, you can always feel stubble. But now, no—I was smooth, with only a strip of hair on the top of my mons veneris, like an arrow pointing down to my hole.

Roderick zoomed in, and stayed zoomed.

I thought I heard him breathing a little harder as he stayed squatting between my legs with the handheld.

I began sliding my middle finger in and out of my pussy, as if I were teasing myself. Not deep.

The fan pushed air at me. The lights lit my skin, made it hot, made my face feel damp and slick.

All of a sudden, I was tired. I just wanted to get on with it, get my pay, get out. I wasn't curious about what it was like to make porn anymore. I was making it. *This is how it feels,* I thought, *to be a porn star.*

The worst part about it was how little I felt about doing it. It was like my emotions were wrapped in bath towels.

"Use the toy," said Roderick.

"Okay," I said.

I reached under the couch and pulled out the black vibrator. There weren't any batteries in it, so it felt unbalanced and light.

"Say something," he said.

I moaned while I tried to think of something to say. I rubbed the vibrator on my pussy to get it wet, so that it wouldn't hurt going in. I was hungry and dehydrated, but I hadn't wanted to drink too much water before the shoot so I wouldn't have to call for a bathroom break. I wondered how much longer the filming would take, and how long I'd have to use the toy. I hoped the smooth plastic wouldn't pinch when I finally inserted it.

"Tell them you want them to fuck you," Roderick said. He brought the camera up close to my pussy. I looked down. Behind the pink lenses, his pupils were dilated.

He was definitely breathing harder.

Maybe filming porn was somehow strenuous for him. It couldn't be that after fifteen years in the adult industry, watching a girl bang herself with a vibrator was still sexy to him. Was it? How could it be? Roderick Saxon could line up a dozen girls and have them all fuck themselves with vibrators in shifts around the clock, if he wanted. Why would he be interested in me doing it in particular? Maybe Roderick was like one of Pavlov's dogs, hardwired to respond to visual stimulus with an erection.

Maybe all men were. *Ugh*. Well, it explained why they spent billions of dollars a year on adult entertainment.

"*Fuck me*," I said. "I want you to fuck me with your big, hard cock. Shove it into my tight, wet pussy."

I pushed the vibrator in. Pulled it out. Pushed it in again.

I felt like occupied space when it was inside me. Unoccupied when it was out. I thought of the tiny bathrooms on airplanes, with the little sliding panel that said if someone was in there or not. Fucking myself with the black vibrator was like sliding that panel back and forth. OCCUPIED. UNOCCUPIED.

I spread my legs, pushing my hips up, as if it were feeling really good.

"Do you want to watch me come?" I asked. It was a rhetorical question.

I was tired of being on my back, so I rearranged myself on the couch, with my ass pointing toward the eye of the big camera.

"Hold on a minute," said Roderick. I heard a click. He had popped the tape out of his handheld, and was labeling a fresh one with his black Sharpie.

"Okay, go," he said.

I arched my back like a cat, shoving my bottom up in the air.

"Go back to the part where you're getting really excited," Roderick said.

I moaned. "Oh, god, yeah, fuck me," I said.

"Can you say that again? But louder—the mike doesn't pick up as well when you're faced away from it."

"*Oh god, yeah, fuck me.*" I put the tip of the vibrator against my pussy. It was awkward. I felt as if I were trying to pin a tail on myself, or put in a tampon from behind. Finally I got the angle right, and pushed it inside.

I moved it in and out, trying to sound more and more excited. I'd gotten wet, so the vibrator wasn't uncomfortable. It was just kind of weird to feel my insides being pushed around, moving to make room for a plastic toy.

Roderick moved around the couch and put the handheld camera up to my face. I looked into the lens. Made eye contact with the men who were going to be watching me later: future men, future viewers.

"*Anal,*" whispered Roderick. "Can you do anal?" He swallowed. "Please?"

I thought about it.

"I guess," I said. "Just a sec."

I put the black toy back under the couch and seized the little red dildo with the flanged base.

"Do you need a break?" asked Roderick.

"No, let's just go," I said.

I didn't even care about the money anymore. I just wanted it to be done so I could leave Roderick Saxon's stupid, expensive condo. I wanted to be home watching TV, wearing my pajama pants and a loose T-shirt. I was weary of the whole thing: tired of talking dirty, sick of putting plastic inside myself, and exhausted from dealing with Roderick, the professional vagina wrangler. If sticking something up my butt could expedite the process of me getting dressed and out the door, I was all for it.

The lace tops of the thigh-high stockings were cutting into my flesh. I knew that when I rolled them off, red lines would show where the elastic had been.

"Do you want lube?" asked Roderick. "I have some upstairs. I can go get it."

"Christ!" I said. "No! Let's just go, okay? Are you ready?"

I had never had anything up my butt before. It seemed like men were always trying to stick their fingers in women's assholes, but I'd never let anyone do that to me. When I felt their fingers tentatively sliding around back there, I always pulled away or said, "No way, I'm not into that," or changed positions so my asshole would be less accessible. Frankly, I had no idea what the big deal was about women's asses, except for the fact that most of us don't want men sticking things in us back there. I thought maybe it was a *challenge and denial* kind of thing—like the more women didn't want it, the more determined men would be to get in, just to feel like they got something over on us or made us feel ridiculous.

Customers at Butterscotch's loved ass talk. Anything that involved them sticking anything in our butts—their fingers, their cocks, their tongues, really anything—seemed to delight them, deeply and primally.

Honestly, though, whenever I talked about ass stuff, I just thought about poop. I mean, poop *comes* from asses. You'd think that would be a turnoff, but apparently, poop didn't matter to the kind of men who enjoyed adult entertainment. They seemed to believe that if nobody mentioned it, poop would just go away and not be a factor anymore.

I spread my knees apart on the couch and surreptitiously rubbed the little red dildo between my legs, to get it wet.

"Fuck my ass," I said. "Fuck it hard. Please, please fuck me. I want to come all over your cock."

I had a little trouble getting the dildo inside my asshole, but I just shoved really hard and it kind of popped in. It felt kind of disgusting, like I was halfway through shitting and had decided to get up with the job only partially done.

I started faking a big, theatrical orgasm. "Oh yes . . . oh yes! Yes! Fuck me!"

I arched my back hard, pushing my ass toward Roderick's camera and wailing like a cat in estrus. "Fuck my ass! I'm coming!"

After I caught my breath, I realized I was still being filmed and decided to go for a second *petite morte*. "Give it to me, come in my hot ass—come with me," I begged.

It was like an encore. I faked a little orgasm, just to be companionable with anyone who hadn't already finished during my prior, larger orgasm.

And I was done. There was no way I was going to go for three. I was tired and hungry, and worst of all, I was dying for a sip of water. I felt like I'd run a marathon or been pummeled by a professional boxer. My back ached and my pussy was sore, and I wanted to rip the tight, uncomfortable lace-banded stockings off my legs as soon as I could. The lace had suddenly become unendurably scratchy and my exhaustion was amplifying the discomfort into torture.

I closed my eyes.

When I opened them, Roderick was turning his cameras off, removing tapes, and gathering clamp lights like they were big, hot daisies. He put them on a table to cool while he wrapped electrical cords back on themselves like ropes.

"That was great, Heidi," he said. "Very hot. You can go ahead and get dressed. We've definitely got enough material for a good scene."

I got up and went to the bathroom. My ass felt slimy. I hoped it was just from my own pussy juice.

I wadded up about half a roll of Roderick's fancy quilted toilet paper and wiped my ass with it. I checked the paper to see if it was tainted with poop, but it wasn't. Thank God. I figured Roderick would have said something if I'd been unclean, but you never knew. Maybe he, too, liked to pretend that poop and asses were two different things, completely foreign to each other.

I couldn't stop wiping. I ended up using up all his fancy toilet paper.

Running water in the sink, I opened Roderick's medicine cabinet to see if he had anything good.

Hemorrhoid cream—yuck. A brand-new toothbrush, still encased in plastic. Crest whitening toothpaste. I hated the whitening stuff—my dentist told me that it just scratched off your tooth enamel. Your teeth ended up browner than ever the longer you used it.

The best thing Roderick had was Tylenol 3, the kind you could buy over the counter in Canada: acetaminophen, caffeine, and codeine.

I flushed the toilet to cover up the sound of me opening the Tylenol, and popped six into my mouth. I chewed them up and swallowed them. Without water, they hurt my throat as they went down. It was like swallowing six little pieces of broken glass.

Dressing quickly, I wadded my panties, white lacy bra, and sundress together and shoved them into my backpack. I crammed my sandals in on top. I didn't care if I wore any of it ever again.

When I came out, Roderick had moved the couch back against the wall and was sitting on it, counting crisp money from out of a bank envelope. He looked up at me quickly.

"I'm calling it two fifty," he said. "I normally pay two for solo stuff, but you did anal, and it was good work, so . . ." He handed me a bunch of twenties and a ten, folded in half. I smiled. Two hundred and fifty dollars was a very good day at Butterscotch's— and I'd just made that in three hours.

"Do you want to work again?" he asked.

"Yeah," I said.

"Do you want something to eat?" Roderick asked me. "I could do with a bite." He looked absurdly hopeful.

Roderick, I just fucked myself in the twat and the ass with toys while you filmed me doing it. I used up all your toilet paper wiping my butt afterward. There is no way I can sit down and eat with you. There is just no fucking way.

"No thanks," I said.

We parted at the door of his apartment. We didn't shake hands.

Three weeks later, I was on the cover of *Fat, Horny Bitches 3*.

I did a few more videos for Roderick Saxon, but that was my first and only Roderick Saxon box cover.

"I Hate Myself for Loving You"— Joan Jett and the Blackhearts

After I did the Roderick Saxon shoot, getting porn work became easier. All I had to do was say I'd worked with Roderick Saxon, and I had instant credibility.

Most of the photographers wanted to know if I'd done a "Roderick Backflush," which was Roderick's signature move. He had an entire page on his website devoted to Backflush footage. The Backflush was when Roderick would get oral sex from the girl and then shoot his cum all over her face in ropes, concentrating on her eyes and mouth. Then the girl would try to smile, and the camera would get really close, and she'd rub the cum all over her face, licking her fingers and sighing. A few of the girls would surreptitiously wipe their eyes first.

Some of the models used their fingers to scoop the cum into their mouths. One model used a metal spoon, scraping the cum off her chin and putting the spoon into her mouth as if the globules of ejaculate on her face were baby food, and she was learning to feed herself. Some of the models just stuck their tongues out and licked the area around their mouths. After the spoon girl, the ones just using their tongues seemed kind of lazy.

Basically the Backflush was about covering the girls' faces in cum, and then having them act like they really liked it, even when it got into their eyes or up their noses.

Some of the girls were really good actresses. They'd roll their heads around and go *"Mmmmmm,"* like the Backflush felt really good, as if the cum tasted delicious. Some of them looked nauseous. The worst ones were the girls who just looked *absent,* like they were a million miles away—like they were just getting though the Backflush so they could get up, towel off, and get their money. When they ate the cum it was like they were trying to get as much of it in their mouths as they could, swallowing it down without tasting it, just to make it disappear. Watching those girls I thought, *I have never needed money that badly.*

Roderick's website let you click on whatever title sounded best to you. There were dozens, including *Fat, Horny Bitches; Here's Cum in Your Eye; Hairy-Boxed Sluts; Black Crackwhore Cocksuckers;* and all the *Pussy Pounder* movies. If you clicked on a title, you saw the box covers of all the movies in the series. I had to admit, Roderick's site was well organized and encyclopedic, as easy to navigate and endlessly archival as the Seattle Public Library's computerized card catalog. Nearly any prurient interest that could possibly exist was represented, and there were entire Roderick Saxon film series made just to cater to that particular interest.

If you selected a series and then clicked on a specific box cover, you could see pictures of all the models in that particular title, plus a larger view of the cover. My pictures were under the series title *Fat, Horny Bitches,* of course; and were indexed under *fat, anal, Heidi, girl next door, dildo, vibrator, white lace,* and *solo action.* I was pretty happy with how I looked. I lay on the couch with my legs in the air, smiling—and then the smaller pictures showed me topless, pulling up my sundress to show my panties. I was surprised at how playful and relaxed I looked.

I saved the URL of my photos and film clips and got used to sending photographers directly to that page on Roderick's site when they asked me what I looked like. When they asked about the Roderick Backflush, I told them, "Absolutely not," and made it clear that I would never do porn that involved male models or any bodily fluids whatsoever. I lost some work over that, but most photographers just sighed and booked with me anyway. After all, I'd been one of Roderick's girls.

I worked for a lot of amateur photographers, websites, and video producers. There was a lot of work in Seattle. I learned who was legitimate and who wasn't, what kind of girls employers liked to use, and what they wanted to see or hear from me. I didn't bother calling the ones who only wanted very skinny or very young models. I went through Adult Help Wanted every week until I could recognize each photographer by his phone number. Roderick advertised a lot.

The weird thing was that the photographers and filmmakers I worked for were considered amateur, but they also paid models on a professional scale and accepted large amounts of money from customers for videotapes, photo sets, website access, and DVDs. I'd always thought amateur porn was just couples filming themselves on their camcorders and posting the results on the Internet because thinking of people watching them have sex turned them on. It turned out that *amateur* just meant any pornography other than the big, expensive DVDs put out by high-rolling companies like Vivid, the kind of movies you saw when you checked in at a hotel and paid extra for "adult features" on the TV. But everything other than that—any models who weren't recognizable names, and any productions that cost under $10,000 to make—was amateur, no matter how professional the shoot was or how much money they were making off their products.

So I became a professional amateur, doing shoot after shoot after shoot. I was an oxymoron—a real, horny girl next door who happened to be a paid, experienced porn star.

I'd take the bus or a cab to the studio with all my costumes and shoes for a particular shoot packed into my backpack. I'd meet the photographer, who would have a designated area where I could change out of my street clothes and put on my makeup. Some of these guys were just hobbyists with studios set up in their homes. Others had fancy commercial spaces, with white curved walls and professional scrims and built-in lighting. A lot of porn producers simply rented hotel rooms and brought their own clamp lights and mikes.

I usually arrived for my shoots in boy-pants and a rock T-shirt, with nothing on my face but sunblock. I'd meet the photographer, get shown to my changing area, and ask him if he had any particular looks in mind for the shoot. If it was a fetish shoot, I'd have whatever garment or footwear he'd previously specified. But my basic costume kit had the white lacy stuff I wore for Roderick, schoolgirl apparel, black dominatrix gear, and a few assorted pairs of stockings, garter belts, thongs, and slips. Depending on the shoot, I could do between one and six costume changes. The ones with a lot of changes were onerous, but I made more money, because they had to pay me for the time it took to change and redo my makeup.

Once I was in costume, I'd sit out in the shooting area and let them do light checks. This was monumentally boring, and I learned to bring a book. I just sat, or stood, and they walked around me, moving lights and making sure that I wasn't in shadow at any angle. I got paid for my time, but it was dull, because all I was doing was serving as a moderately lustrous object for the photographer to light. A lot of them took hours getting their lights hung and arranging reflectors that looked like silver umbrellas or aluminum-foil-covered panels. I learned to like the photographers who took the time to bounce their lights off diffusers, because that was less hot than having the lights pointed directly at me, and the end result was more flattering.

I learned that overlighting is the poor man's airbrush: Most women look better in photos if they're lit so much that their skin washes out a bit. I learned to request strong, even light on my face. The clamp lights felt hot and terrible, as if I were sticking my face onto the tanning bed at Butterscotch's, but the white light burned away every flaw I had—the lines, the dark circles under my eyes, the blemishes, everything. I ended up looking like a movie star. In every shoot I figured out where my strongest light was and turned to face it, like a sunflower. It was nice when the photographers put a fan behind the light to lift my hair and give the pictures some movement. The breeze felt good on my skin and kept me from sweating too much.

I learned to pose with only one thing to sit or lean against, like a chair or a bed. If nothing was available to sit on or bend over, I'd use the wall as support for some of my poses. I'd move from frontal poses featuring my breasts to rear positions that showcased my butt, then back again. As I went back and forth between boobs and ass, I'd strip down and get progressively more explicit. I felt like a chunk of salmon on a grill, being flipped again and again.

Eventually I'd end up topless and bottomless, though I nearly always kept my stockings and shoes on. Then I'd do spread stuff, which meant opening my legs and using my fingers to pull my puss apart. I'm not sure why the spread shots were so popular, but it seemed like every single photographer wanted them. I thought it made my pussy look like sashimi. *Spread* also included ass stuff, where I used my hands to pull my ass cheeks apart so the photographer could take pictures of my asshole. I found out that mine was considered very attractive: It was pink instead of brown, and pleasingly virginal in appearance.

The first time a photographer complimented my asshole, the absurdity of it all washed over me in waves and all I could think was how incredibly surreal my life had become—that I was in a hotel room fielding a polite compliment about my anus, the way some women say graceful thank-yous to comments about their lovely eyes or hair. Soon the compliments were frequent enough that I developed asshole pride, as if it were my secret weapon. I learned to frame my actual hole with my hands, as if I were inviting the viewer to come partake.

My routine from there on out was pretty clear-cut. From the spread poses I'd move on to fake fingerbanging. I learned to bend my fingers and put my knuckles up against my puss or ass to make it look like my fingers were inside me. There was no reason to really insert them. The bent-finger method photographed really well, even in extreme close-up, and photographers and viewers couldn't tell the difference. It spared me wear and tear inside, too.

From there, I'd move on to toy stuff. First the pussy, then the butt. Again, the fact that I was willing to perform object penetration in my back door got me bunches of repeat bookings. For me, sticking a toy in my butt was no different than sticking one in my pussy. Neither one felt good, but if I did anal, I'd make more money and get more work.

After toy penetration, I was done with the shoot. I could clean the lube off myself, dress, and go home. I preferred cash, but I'd take a check from someone I'd worked with before, or who came highly recommended to me by another model or photographer. I usually made $100–$150 per hour, and most shoots lasted from two to four hours. The proofs belonged to the photographer. I usually never saw the results of the shoot, though most of them were available online. After I'd checked out Roderick's site, I was just never that curious: I assumed I pretty much looked like any other porn model. I never worried about being recognized in real life because I looked so different on film with my wigs, heavy makeup, and body-modifying costumes. What the viewers wanted—a tall, curvy, dirty-talking babe willing to take it in the ass—ceased to exist the second the cameras were turned off. It was easy to compartmentalize, because the brazen girl I was on film was so completely fabricated.

After the first few shoots I started bringing my own toys in a waterproof plastic bag. If you didn't bring your own, you were at the mercy of what they had, and those toys tended to be really large. I made a habit of putting lube on my pussy before penetrating myself with a toy, because the lube photographed as "wetter" than my own internal moisture. I learned from other models that when doing a toy shoot, the best time to be photographed was not as the toy was going *in*, but as it was being pulled *out*. That way, my labia weren't pushed back into the vagina by the toy; they were instead wrapped *around* the toy, giving the appearance of a larger toy in a smaller hole.

I learned to relax my inner muscles so the toys wouldn't hurt. If I clenched up, the toys were horribly uncomfortable, since they were unyielding, hard plastic. I took breaks and breathed deeply to make sure I wouldn't involuntarily react to the plastic invasion of my internal space by clamping down.

I learned to squirt hair conditioner on my pussy and my butt to make fake cum. I used Kiehl's Leave-In Hair Conditioner because it was nice and thick and wouldn't melt or get runny under the hot lights. It even smelled good, making my stripe of pubic hair lush, fragrant, and soft.

I continued to work my regular four shifts a week at Butterscotch's, and shot porn about twice a week. I was busy. A few Butterscotch's customers recognized me as Heidi, the anal-toy-loving slut. I told the customers who'd seen me in *Fat, Horny Bitches* that I'd done the Roderick Saxon Backflush off camera, and that it had turned me on so much I'd come in my panties. They loved hearing about how salty and delectable Roderick's cum was, and how delighted I'd been when he'd emptied his big, hairy balls all over my face. It became abundantly clear to me that the Roderick Saxon Backflush was a way for men to delight in another man's semen without thinking of themselves as gay.

Chapter 3
Pussy Sweatshop

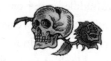

"Voodoo" — Godsmack

The New Year brought constant, pissing rain, and mud, and continual darkness.

At Butterscotch's, we huddled in the lounge wrapped in blankets, circled around our campfire, the TV. We slept a lot, curled up on the couch or in blanket pallets on the floor. Every so often the door would *beeeeeeeep,* and we'd look at each other, rumpled and hazy from napping in the dry glow of the electrical space heater, and one of us would go out to attempt to corral the person in the lobby into a show. Our shows became spastic and lackluster. The lingerie rooms were cold, and we wanted to get our sessions over with quickly, so we could get back to the TV and our nests of blankets.

I didn't bother dancing or being seductive anymore. I just knelt between the customers' spread legs and rubbed the triangle of fabric over my crotch, about two inches above my actual clitoris. I fake-masturbated and fake-came, telling the customers how horny I was, and how much I wanted to watch them shoot their loads onto their own stomachs. It was a rare moment when I felt compelled to be more creative.

I was bored. My shows were rote.

Plus, I was sick of getting touched. They weren't supposed to touch us and we made that clear, but every now and again a customer would attempt to breach the invisible wall between us, grabbing for my skin with slick, smelly fingers. Getting touched by them was humiliating and disgusting, like being brushed with dog shit. I had to be constantly on the lookout for sneaky hands, or customers attempting to point their cocks at me. When they did try to touch or point, I had to deal with the situation immediately, roaring *Sit down, Don't touch me,* or *Point your shit* away *from me.* If they didn't comply, their shows were over. The constant vigilance was exhausting.

I became curious about other work available in Seattle. I was still modeling regularly, but I wanted to branch out, to learn more.

I noticed an ad in Adult Help Wanted for a place called Eros Galaxy. They needed models for part-time live work. Most of the other ads that week were Roderick Saxon's. He was looking for chubby girls again. My guess was that he was probably casting for *Fat, Horny Bitches 4.*

"Do you know anything about Eros Galaxy?" I asked Crystal. She was the Zagat of the local sex industry: She'd been working in Seattle for over ten years, and if she hadn't worked in a particular establishment, she'd hired girls who had.

Over the months, I had come to realize that in the sex industry—where the workers who supply the labor have very little redress for unfair treatment—word of mouth was essential. Our status as "independent contractors" meant we were isolated; we were rogue workers without any professional support or organized clout. It wasn't like we could go to Labor and Industries and expect any of our grievances to be taken seriously.

"The peep show?" Crystal was rolling black lace stockings up her legs. The lace looked scratchy.

"Yeah, the peep show, I guess," I said. "I'm thinking of picking up a few shifts over there. Do you know how it works?"

"Shit," Crystal said. "Going to the peeps is like going to jail."

Jail? "How so?"

"It's a pussy sweatshop. The other girls can be mean, too— they're competitive. They don't take turns there the way we do here." She looked at me. "You know it's nude work, right?"

I did. It said *nude* right in the ad. And *no contact,* which meant no slimy fingers. That sounded good.

Crystal clipped her scratchy-looking lace stockings to her garter belt. Two clips in the front, two on each side. I hated garter belts—they always pulled down and cut into my waist, and it seemed like they never kept my stockings up anyway.

A pussy sweatshop. Like going to jail.

"Can you make money there?" I asked.

"Yeah," said Crystal. "It's really different than here, though. You have to be—" Crystal stopped. "Well, you have to be tough. I guess *tough* is the word."

I felt pretty tough.

I determined to go to Eros Galaxy on my next day off, just to check it out. It was exciting to think about learning another aspect of the adult industry. It had been a while since I'd felt challenged by my work. A pussy sweatshop?

Well, bring it on, I thought. I wanted to know it all, to learn everything. If I *could* do it, why *shouldn't* I? I didn't have far to fall. I did, in fact, know my shit.

Besides, I was used to being nude for photo and video work. I had my secret weapon, my beautiful, rosy, virginal asshole. That killed, nearly every time.

From the outside, Eros Galaxy looked like a dirty bookstore. Painted boards covered the windows, blocking the store's interior from view, and every board featured an evocative, vaguely raunchy-sounding sentence fragment like SEATTLE'S HOTTEST ADULT or XXX THEATER or LIVE NUDE MODELING.

I pushed open the door and went in.

In front of me were a long flight of steps and a sign that read ARCADE. An arrow pointed up. I heard music upstairs, and a porno soundtrack. "Oh, oh, oh, fuck me," said the lady on the soundtrack. She sounded like she was doing my lingerie show. She was breathing too hard, though. She sounded corny—her moans and all that panting. Hyperventilation wasn't sexy. I tried to keep my moaning and audible breathing to a minimum in my sessions—a real woman wouldn't gasp for breath like that unless she were in an iron lung.

When I got to the top of the stairs, a counter was to my left, and to my right a row of doors faced the counter. A tired old gay guy with stainless steel plugs in his earlobes was behind the counter. His head was shaved, his eyebrows plucked bare past the middle of each arch so they pointed up like Spock's. Was he wearing rouge?

"What can I do for you today, sweetie?" he asked in an exquisitely bored, nasal drone. It was as if he were asking a question and saying *I couldn't care less* at the same time.

"I saw the ad. I want to work," I said.

The carpets underfoot were plush, but the place stank. The stink differed from Butterscotch's—Eros Galaxy's odor had more bleach in it, like the smell of a community center swimming pool. Underneath the bleach smell was the thick, familiar scent of the rank things that come from men's bodies: cum, farts, saliva, sweat, shit. These places were like public latrines to them. They came in, spewed their filth, and walked away from their own foulness, lighter and freer.

Sex work, it occurred to me, was much like toilet training. It was certainly way more about *their* bodies than it was about *ours*. We were paid to manage, direct, and tolerate their waste, ignoring the stench and cooing over their various evacuations, like erotic bathroom attendants. A girl who could make a customer feel good about dumping his sexual feculence in her presence was a girl who made money, not the girl with the biggest tits or the best ass. Our looks were beside the point.

I had regulars who saw me again and again for sessions, and they weren't even interested in my body at all. They looked at my tits and ass perfunctorily, of course, but ultimately what they wanted was encouragement. They loved to hear me say, *Jerk that cock for me. Come for me. Fuck your ass for me. Yes. Yes yes yes.* It was my words and my approving manner—not my body or the sleazy costumes I wore—that normalized my customers' infantile urges to display the physical functions that are usually considered private.

Eros Galaxy certainly smelled like a public toilet. My nose and throat were beginning to burn from the bleach aroma.

"You ready to work?" said the counterman. "You got your stuff?"

"Yeah," I said. I had a costume and makeup in my backpack, as well as baby wipes and a liter of water.

"You dance before?"

"Yeah," I said. "Butterscotch's."

"You girls suck dick there," the counterman said. It wasn't a question. At least he finally sounded remotely engaged. He stared at me. He was definitely wearing mascara: His eyes looked like cheap doll eyes with painted lines around them for lashes.

I looked into his foxy, mean little face. His mouth was queenishly puckered, like an old lady's change purse. It was drawn up tight like an anus.

"I don't suck dick," I said. "None of my friends suck dick." I kept my voice low.

The counterman and I stared at each other, like we were having a showdown. Our eyes were fighting each other. *This town's not big enough for both of us, Sheriff.* I tried to make my eyes narrow and hard, like a gunslinger's.

I thought, *Look at Quentin Crisp, calling* me *a cocksucker.*

"I'm here to work," I said again.

The counterman finally looked away, rummaging around below and coming up with a crumpled, xeroxed form.

"Fill this out," he droned. He acted like we hadn't even been fighting. I figured that meant I'd won.

Name, Address—I made both up.

Phone number. My cell.

Washington State ID number. I wrote it down, jumbling the final four digits. It was none of their business. I had no idea who these people were, and the only Eros Galaxy employee I'd ever met had just accused me of prostitution. *Fuck you, Eros,* I thought. *How about this? You can suck* my *dick.*

Social Security number. 666-66-6666. It wasn't like I was eligible for health benefits, or workers' comp.

Stage name: After a moment of deliberation, I wrote *Holiday.* The name seemed like an utterly dippy and ridiculous choice, a contemptuous fuck-you to anyone fantasizing about me being anything other than a paid performer. I was sick of my customers pretending that I performed sex work innocently, out of some mistake.

If they wanted fake, I'd give them fake.

I didn't expect to work at Eros very long, anyway. The place seemed dead. Since I'd arrived, not a single customer had come up the stairs.

"Stranglehold"— Ted Nugent

Once I'd filled out the application, the counterman shoved it into the register and took me down a dimly lit hall, past the booths facing the counter. We walked past a series of windows, set into the hallway at about eye level. Some of the windows had curtains pulled across them imperfectly. The curtains were shoddy and flammable looking, like the little privacy drapes that never completely block the sun from your eyes when you ride on the wrong side of the Greyhound bus.

Two of the windows didn't have stained fabric pulled across them, though, and I could see into them. The undraped windows opened onto plain, plastic cubes about big enough to sit in, but definitely not big enough to stand in without stooping. There were doors inside the cubes facing the windows—tiny little half-size dwarf doors, like shutters. The cubes were mostly empty, though one had a dirty-looking blanket on its plastic floor.

It was a human-size dog kennel. It was like those cages at the animal shelter where you could look at the sad, hopeful dogs that were going to get killed if you didn't take them home. The only things missing were a few bowls of dog chow and dirty water, and maybe a couple of crusty chew toys. But I was pretty sure that the cubes were for women, not dogs.

Next to each window was a doorway with a curtain in it, like a shower stall. The curtains were made of red velvet, syphilitic with cigarette burns. They didn't go all the way to the floor, so if you stood in the booth, anyone passing by could see your feet. I peeked through a gap in one of the curtains and saw a box of Kleenex on the floor, and a complicated-looking wall grille that looked like the front of a change machine. Next to the change machine was a telephone handset. The curtain itself smelled strongly of piss.

I followed the counterman past the plastic windows and around a corner to an unmarked door. He selected one key from a huge bundle and turned it in the lock. "Go on in," he said. "Nobody showed up to work today, so it's all yours."

He put his keys back into his pocket. "Lazy bitches," he said. "Are you lazy?"

"Me?" I said. "No, I'm not lazy."

He snorted.

We were clearly in the dressing room. Makeup tables stood against two of the walls—with real, movie-star-style round lightbulbs around the mirrors, I noticed, instead of the Christmas lights we had at Butterscotch's. There was a mini fridge next to one of the tables. I could see a small bathroom off the main room, also lit with frosted bulbs.

Three half-size doors along one wall of the dressing room led to the plastic cubicles. The doors started at waist level, and went up a little bit past my head. The counterman went over and opened one.

"Ta-da," he said. I could see that in order to get into the plastic cube I'd have to jump or crawl up, scrambling gracelessly through the midget-size door and up onto the plastic floor of the cube. There were no steps. It seemed like a bad design to me.

And I was tall! I wondered what the shorter girls did. Maybe they had to pull chairs over from the makeup tables to get into their boxes.

"You do your private shows here, in the booths," the counterman said.

"How much are they?"

The counterman sighed. "I'm not gonna tell you how to do your job, sweetie," he said. "Get whatever you can get. The customers put their money through the automated slot, just like they're buying a Coke or something. That gives them their time. They tip into the slots, too. The house gets half."

"Half my tips?"

"Half of everything. And you pay twenty dollars a shift stage fee to work. That comes out of your end, not ours. On top of the half." The counterman stared at me challengingly.

I didn't say anything.

"Once they're in the booth, make them pick up the phone. That way they can hear you. And don't forget to close the curtains in your booth so you're not doing your show for everyone in the hallway.

"What name are you going by?" he asked me.

"Holiday," I said.

He rolled his eyes.

"Like, uh, Judy Holliday?" I said. "And the Madonna video?" *And the tacky-ass Holiday Inn down the street, with AstroTurf for a lawn?*

"Whatever," he said. "We've had far, far stupider names, I suppose. Did you write that on your application?"

"Yeah," I said.

He sighed. "I'm Stewie," he said.

"I'm pleased to meet—"

"Look," he said, "we get half of everything in the booths. We get everything onstage, but you keep your tips there. They tip through the slots there."

"Where's the stage?"

Stewie pointed past the cubicle doors, toward a few carpeted steps. I noticed a freestanding rack of lockers near the stairs. Some of them were padlocked. Most of them looked like they'd been broken into: The metal doors were warped away from their frames like melted salvage from a house fire. Judging from the gouges in the metal around a few of the locks, it was also possible that the doors had been pried back with screwdrivers. There were stickers and Magic Markered graffiti all over them, as well as violent-looking punctures and dents. They were pretty much the least secure lockers I'd ever seen.

"Bring a padlock if you want a locker. Or not," said Stewie, shrugging. "Some girls just bring everything they need, every day."

"That's understandable," I said.

"The stage is right up those steps," said Stewie. He looked at me. "No penetration onstage. That'll get us shut down."

"Penetration?"

"No fingers or toys in your hoo-hoo or ass," he said. "Onstage."

"Okeydokey." I hadn't brought any toys. I made a mental note to bring some next time. I had a small army of different sex toys that I used for shoots, so it wasn't like I'd have to buy any new ones.

"When you have a customer for stage, I'll try to flash the stage lights for you, so you'll know to come over. But sometimes I don't have time to do that, so you have to keep checking your stage windows to see if there's anyone there."

"Okay." I had no idea what Stewie was talking about.

"So, get dressed and get to work. If you have any questions, come out and ask. But try to stay back here—we really don't like girls in the front."

You really don't like girls anywhere, *do you?* I thought. "Okay," I said.

"You're late for the 10:00 AM shift. It's noon now. You're on till 7:00 PM. There's another shift from 7:00 PM till whenever. Don't be late, or we charge you twenty bucks on top of your stage. No leaving early, ever."

"Okay," I said.

"Three no-shows means you're fired."

I nodded.

"All right," said Stewie. "Holiday, right? I'll go put your name into the front booth, so just work out of that one today."

"Thank you," I said.

Stewie's chapped lips quivered.

"You're welcome," he snapped. "Now get dressed. We've already had some calls. You need to be ready for customers."

He stomped out of the dressing room. I heard the door lock behind him.

I was a little affronted by Stewie's relentless hostility, but he was such a weird little troll, with his bald head and his stretched-out earlobes and his Sunset Boulevard makeup, that it was hard to take too much offense. I was pleased to have the place to myself— I could figure out how to make money without being sabotaged or misled by other girls, and I could read, undisturbed, between customers. By the time I had to share dressing room, stage, and box space with the other Eros workers, I'd be at the top of my game, with my own established routines and the beginnings of my own clientele. I was eager to get started, to carve out my own territory and figure out the most effective ways to maximize my hustle, working within the given parameters.

Like going to jail, I thought. *Well, bring it on.* I was ready.

"Living Dead Girl"— Rob Zombie

I went into the bathroom and found some Lysol and paper towels. I cleaned off one of the makeup tables, then put my backpack on top of it and changed into costume.

I'd brought an old standard for luck—an ensemble that had always made me money at Butterscotch's, consisting of a red lace bra, matching red thong panties, red stay-up thigh-high fishnet stockings, and a red satin slip. The customers loved my red set dearly and often requested that I wear it for them. All that red was probably exciting. It certainly was undeniably whorish. I'd learned that to most men, elegance and subtlety were far less stirring than the semblance of blatant professional availability.

Most men claimed they were looking for a classy, dignified woman—a *lady*—but when it came right down to who actually got paid, the depraved trailer trash slut won over the debutante every single time.

There was a rip in one of my fishnet stockings. I made sure to turn it around, so the rip appeared on the back of my leg, instead of the front.

I strapped on the red patent leather stiletto heels I'd bought specifically to go with my red costume set. They added six inches to my height and made my legs look thinner, plus they were so shiny they looked like licked cherry lollipops. Men loved them, and begged to mouth them. Occasionally I'd let a domination client suck on the heels.

I put on lipstick and used pressed powder on my nose, forehead, and chin. Then I tucked my hair back under a nylon wig cap and put on an old blond wig I'd paid Viva $20 for. It was platinum blond and didn't match my eyebrows, but I liked the way I looked in it: cheap and trashy. It smelled like Viva. I thought of the cedar chips people put in their closets to keep moths away.

Looking in the mirror, I was pleased to meet Holiday. She looked like a real good time.

The "stage" at Eros Galaxy was more like a carpeted closet. It was small—maybe eight feet long and five feet deep. There were full-length mirrors against the back wall, making me feel like a plastic ballerina doll in a music box. Opposite the mirrors was a row of tinted windows where I guessed the customers would appear, when they came. Next to each window was a tip slot.

Vertical grip bars were mounted on the sides of each window so you could squat, hold onto the bars, and lean back, to show your girl-parts to the customers more effectively. The ingenuity of the vertical bars impressed me. I pictured stirrups on either side of the windows for our feet, so we could rest comfortably with our knees lifted and apart. I wondered if some day the management would simply hand out disposable speculums to the customers so they could see all the way up to our cervixes.

Right across from the stage was the front box, the one Stewie had assigned me. I peeked in.

My box was lit by one very bright lightbulb, like a life-size Easy-Bake oven. The plastic surface of the walls and floor looked unclean, covered with shoe scuff marks, long, stray hairs, and a few dried puddles of what I hoped was just old lubricant. I went back to the dressing room for Lysol and paper towels. Before cleaning my cubicle, I folded a few paper towels to fashion a shade for the lightbulb, dimming and diffusing the light a little bit. I made a mental note to check the towels frequently so they wouldn't singe from the bulb's heat.

I remembered the sound of the door locking behind Stewie and thought of the Triangle Shirtwaist Company. One hundred and forty-six seamstresses died—most of them immigrants desperate for a better life—because a fire started in the sweatshop where they sewed, and they couldn't get out. Those ladies were martyrs for labor. Their deaths meant something, and led to improvement in working conditions for the poor. But if my lightbulb set the paper towels on fire, would anyone care about one dead stripper?

I couldn't count on Stewie to save me. He'd probably throw gasoline on the flames.

I tried not to think of all the STDs one could catch from working nude in such unsanitary conditions. Hepatitis! Herpes! I made a mental note to squat—not sit—when my panties were off. The last thing I wanted was to rub my girl-parts against the same plastic floor all the other strippers had rubbed *their* girl-parts on. Did the health department even know about Eros Galaxy? I mean, they visited restaurants to make sure that employees had bleach buckets, and that everyone washed their hands before handling food. Why would they let an establishment offer us such dangerous, disease-promoting working conditions? Was it just that they didn't care? You'd think Eros Galaxy wouldn't want their girls getting sick from each other, at the very least.

But the evidence to the contrary was inarguable. The booth was rancid. The paper towels kept coming up brown from all the accumulated filth. I felt dizzy from the Lysol fumes, but the squalor only made me more determined. I was going to make a clean, safe little home for myself in my plastic box, and I was going to learn all the ins and outs of working fully nude behind glass. What kind of tough girl would I be if I let a little dirt scare me away from a venue that intrigued me so much? The money was almost beside the point—I wanted to make as much as I could, of course, but my motivation was primarily the rush of learning a new system, adding another layer to my expertise in adult work. I couldn't wait for my first customer. What kind of man would come here to jerk off behind a smelly velvet curtain while staring through a window at a live, naked girl in a plastic kennel? It was so sick I couldn't stand not to be part of it, at least for a little while.

After I finished wiping down my booth, I got my coat from the dressing room. I laid it down on the floor of the booth, so I could sit on that instead of on the bare plastic. I figured the coat could always be dry-cleaned. My booth smelled strongly of disinfectant, but at least it was less overtly filthy than it had been. I wondered who had worked in my booth before me. Whoever she was, she'd smelled like old farts, coconut oil, and menthol cigarettes. The next girl in my booth would think I smelled like a can of bathroom cleanser. I wasn't sure which was worse.

I crawled into my cube and sat cross-legged on my coat with my back against the wall, facing the window where customers could put their money in and watch me perform. It was a little claustrophobic—I could touch both walls easily from where I sat, and if I stretched, I could touch the ceiling. I breathed deeply to calm myself.

The lightbulb's heat baked the top of my wig. Was the hair fiber flammable? I used my finger to scratch my damp, sweaty scalp, which was trapped under my matted real hair and the nylon wig cap. The blond bangs hung in my eyes and stuck to my forehead, glued down with perspiration. How did Lenore and Viva wear their wigs and look so cool and comfortable? Was there some kind of trick to it? Did I just have an unusually hot head?

I noticed a button to my upper right, next to the window. When I pressed it, the shade went up a few inches. Pressing the button again made the shade come back down. Under the button, and connected through the wall of the booth to the bill collector on the other side, was an LCD display. Red letters on a black digital field spelled HOLIDAY across a scrolling marquee. I was absurdly touched.

It occurred to me that somebody had *designed* this entire system, actually drew up the plans and measured everything and made sure it all worked, just like any other automated system: the boxes, the bill-collecting grilles, the automatic curtain—everything. *What kind of maniac would dream up the most efficient way to create a zoo of living, breathing women in plastic cubes?* I wondered. Did that person also design coin-operated Laundromats, or gas chambers? It was the efficiency that was sinister.

I looked out the side window, feeling like a bag of Cheetos in a vending machine, just sitting and waiting to be picked.

Every now and again, a customer passed by, literally window-shopping. Whenever I saw one I smiled invitingly, but usually they avoided my eyes and just walked right past. It was frustrating—they were out there, and I was behind glass. I couldn't sell them a show the way I could at Butterscotch's, because they couldn't *hear* me. I had to figure out some way to get them into the shower stall next to my window so I could get them to pick up the phone handset, so I could convince them to buy a show. Just sitting there wasn't getting me paid—and I owed the house $20 already. I had to do something.

The next time a man passed by my box, I knocked on the glass loudly. He looked up, startled.

"*Hey!*" I shouted. "Go in there!" I pointed to the curtained booth next to my cube.

The man looked confused. He was short and neatly dressed, in Dockers and a polo shirt.

"*Go in there!*" I rapped on the glass harder, and pointed again. "*Go in!*"

He did. He was behind the window with the two layers of glass and the automated curtain. I banged on that window. "Now, *pick up the phone!*" I screamed.

I heard static. He'd picked up!

"... Hello?" he said.

"Hi, baby," I said. "Can you hear me all right?"

"... Yeah," he said.

"Do you want a show?" I asked.

"How much?"

I honestly didn't know.

"What's it worth to you to see my hot wet pussy, baby?" I asked.

There was a long pause.

"I don't know," said the man. We both pondered the question.

"I'm so horny," I said. "I want to make myself come just for you."

"I have twenty bucks," he said. "Is that enough?"

Twenty bucks. Split half and half with the house, the way Stewie said the money was split for booth shows. My half, the ten, would be half of the twenty bucks I owed the house.

Fuck. How was I supposed to make any money here? It was nuts: If I did the show, I'd still end up owing the house ten bucks.

But owing ten was better than owing twenty.

"Put the twenty into the bill collector, baby," I said.

I heard a grinding purr as the machine ate the man's bill. Once the money was absorbed, the curtain in between the two panes of glass rose slowly. My stomach lurched.

Remember to pull the curtain so you're not doing your show for everyone in the hallway. I yanked the hallway window curtain closed.

The customer and I faced each other, staring at each other through a double pane of industrial glass. He held the phone against his ear with his shoulder. His hands were already at his crotch, fumbling. He took his cock out through his fly, then spat into one hand.

"You like that?" he said.

I got on my knees, on my coat. I spread my legs wide and pulled up my slip.

"Look how wet you made me," I said.

"I want to see that pussy," he said.

I was a little amused. He'd been so shy! I'd had to bang on the glass and scream just to get him into my booth! And now that he had his dick out, he was Mr. Confident.

I got on all fours and pointed my ass toward him.

My booth filled up with the sound of his breathing.

"I want to see that pussy," he said again.

I stood in a crouch and removed my panties. Then I got back down on all fours, on my coat.

I spread my knees wide apart, supported myself on one hand, and reached back with the other hand to spread my ass cheeks apart in an old, familiar move.

"I'm gonna come!" he said.

"Come on my ass, baby," I said.

I looked back at him just in time to see him spray my window with pearly strings of semen.

He squeezed the last few drops out, then tucked his spent cock back into his Dockers. "Thanks," he muttered into the phone. Then he hung up the handset and left the booth.

After a few minutes the curtain came down, so I didn't have to keep looking at the ejaculatory fluid on the window as it trickled down the glass in little rivulets.

I put my panties back on. My heart was pounding.

I felt lifted—energized. Working at the peeps was so much easier than working at Butterscotch's! All I had to do was show my girl-parts, just like doing a porn shoot. Big deal! I didn't have to deal with being grabbed, or having to clean up used washcloths afterward, or anything. No fuss, no muss. It was like sex work deconstructed into its most representative parts: You pay me, I show you my pussy. It was brilliantly postmodern.

I didn't even have to be particularly inventive with my dirty talk—the girl-parts were the bottom line. By showing them, I was cutting out 90 percent of my work.

I opened the curtain that allowed potential customers to see me from the hall. A man was waiting outside. He was black and husky, and wore an orange reflective vest. I figured he was a construction worker on his lunch break. He looked uncomfortable in the hallway. I wondered if he'd heard my first customer breathing hard and saying *I'm gonna come.* The construction worker had to have heard my customer jerking off—he'd been right outside the booth. I imagined an Olympic torch relay, the first man handing the second one the box of Kleenex as they passed each other.

"Hey!" I yelled. I pointed at the stall next to my booth. "Go in there!"

He did.

"Pick up the phone!" I shouted, slapping the glass with the palm of my hand.

We negotiated briefly. I agreed to "masturbate" for $40.

When the shade went up between us, I was relieved to note that most of the previous customer's semen had either dried, run off, or become clear. The window was a little blurry where the spray had shot and dripped, but it wasn't too apparent.

I got on my back and spread my legs, bracing the heels of my red pumps against the upper corners of the box. Instead of taking off my panties I just pulled them aside. Then I bent my fingers and tapped my knuckles against my labia, as if I were penetrating myself.

While I moaned "Fuck me!" I did the math. Forty divided by two was $20, and I still owed $10 to the house. That meant I made $10, free and clear, off this show.

"Get your pussy closer," begged the customer.

I scooted closer to the glass and used my fingers to spread myself apart. The customer put his face up to the glass at pussy level. Then he started to lick, flicking his tongue against the glass like a lizard.

I couldn't believe it. Couldn't he taste the previous customer's cum?

"Yeah, lick my pussy," I said. "Lick it real good, baby."

The little darting movements of his tongue became longer and wetter. At every lick I shrieked and thrashed around, as if he were actually licking my pussy instead of cum-covered glass. He licked the glass until it was no longer hazy.

I thought of the word *punishment*.

Was I punishing him?

Did I want him to be punished?

But I wasn't doing anything, was I? I was just spreading my legs and showing my parts, being a "live nude model," as per my job description. He was the one choosing to lick the Eros Galaxy peep show booth glass—I wasn't making him do it.

But why did it feel so good, so *right,* to watch one customer unknowingly lick up another customer's semen?

After all, I was doing sex work because I wanted to. Nobody was forcing me. Right? Why punish the men who paid me for my work? Wasn't it all fair and square?

Why didn't I warn him, *stop* him?

Instead I couldn't stop laughing. I covered my laughter by pretending to come.

The glass licker finished himself off, pumping into his own hand while he administered a few final tongue-swats to the glass. Then he licked his own semen off his palm and grinned at me.

Oral fixation, I thought.

"Bye-bye!" I said, waving my whole hand like a child.

He waved back and left the booth, walking off jauntily. His orange vest shimmered in the low light.

I was stunned by our mutual depravity.

As I opened my curtain and scanned the hall for potential customers, I realized that yes, I hated them. I hated them. I hated their flat gaze and their poking fingers and the disgusting things they wanted to do. I hated their eyes and their hands and their mouths and their cocks. I hated that they came to places like Butterscotch's and Eros Galaxy. I hated the way they picked out women as if we were inanimate hunks of skin and meat and bone, and then satisfied themselves in front of us without any shame at all. I hated the fact that they didn't want any more from us than our parts splayed in front of them. It was demented.

Did they think we were robots? Did they think we couldn't *see* them?

Punishment. Yes.

The lights onstage went on and off, as if someone were flipping a light switch up and down. They flashed for a few seconds, then stayed on. I remembered Stewie telling me he'd flash the lights if a customer went into one of the front booths for a stage show. One must have arrived. My first stage! I reminded myself not to fake penetration. No toys, no fingers.

I crawled out of my box and walked past the steps to the stage. It felt lovely to be able to stand up and move freely again.

Grabbing a quick glance in the mirrors behind me, I straightened my wig. It had fallen forward a bit during my booth show, giving me the appearance of having a shortened, Cro-Magnon forehead. I pulled it back on my head.

I heard the ratcheting sound of money being worked through a bill collector and tried to guess which window would have the customer behind it.

Suddenly, a window blinked on. There was no curtain: The stage window just went from black and opaque to see-through, all of a sudden. It reminded me of polarized sunglasses. Behind the stage window were a man's head and shoulders. One shoulder twitched as his hand jackhammered at his crotch.

I remembered Stewie telling me that the house took all the bill-collected money onstage, but that we could keep the cash that went through our tip slots. There was no way I was going to be masturbated to without being paid.

I went down on my knees and called through the narrow slot.

"Hey, honey, how are you doing?"

He didn't answer.

"Put some money through this slot, okay baby?"

He didn't make a move, except to continue his mechanical, one-armed jerking.

"Hey!" I said. "Put some goddamned money through the slot, jackass!"

The customer jumped, startled. He stopped yanking at his cock and leaned hesitantly toward the tip slot on his side.

"How much?" he said.

"Give me—uh—" I didn't know. At Butterscotch's, all the prices were set. Here at Eros, it seemed like we could make up whatever prices we wanted. I loved that I could tell the customers what to pay me, and that I was free to accept or reject any counteroffers. It was total pussy anarchy, a labial free-for-all.

"Give me twenty bucks," I said. "Right through here." I knocked at the tip slot so he would know to put the money through it, instead of in the bill collector. Eros had already made enough money off me today.

There had to be ways to beat the system. So far I'd made $10 from a total of three customers. True, I'd paid off my house fee, but at Butterscotch's I was used to making at least $20 per customer, plus tips—and that wasn't even going nude. Granted, the volume at Eros seemed higher and the work was easier, but still—maybe Crystal would know a few hustles for this kind of work. I made a mental note to ask her.

Until then, I'd do the best I could to extort money from the customers using intimidation. That seemed to work pretty well, actually—if you yelled at them, they'd do what you said. Behind glass, being sweet and nice got you ignored.

After all, I hadn't gotten any customers in my booth until I started knocking on the glass and *ordering* them to go in. And I'd had to yell at my stage customer to get him to stop jacking off and start negotiating my tip.

Apparently, most customers were curs: If you acted like the alpha dog, they'd drop their tails and obey reflexively.

"I said, *give me twenty dollars.* Now."

"I got ten."

"Give me ten, then. Hurry up."

He slid the crumpled ten-dollar bill through the tip slot.

I removed my slip, took my bra off, and shook my boobs in the window. The customer started jerking himself again.

"If you wanna see my pussy, it's five more dollars," I said. I was getting used to talking through the slot.

"All I had was that ten!"

"Yeah?" I said. *Punish.* "Too bad, sugar pie! No pussy for you today!"

At that, his window became suddenly opaque. He hadn't put in enough money.

I heard another bill being put into the machine. His window winked back on.

"At least put your tits up to the glass," he said, masturbating furiously.

"I thought all you had was that ten, bitch," I said. I laughed and pressed my breasts against my side of the glass for a moment, thinking of how distorted they probably looked on his side, the way human faces turn into pig masks when you press your nose and cheeks against a window. I pulled away from the glass just in time to watch my customer squirt semen against the front of his booth.

I grabbed the ten-dollar bill and walked offstage, without saying *thanks* or *goodbye.*

You have to be—well, tough.

Like going to jail.

I tucked the bill into my backpack, and went back to my box. Every time someone passed by, I smacked the glass until it trembled.

By 7:00 PM my throat was raw from yelling through glass windows and tip slots. But between the money I'd collected onstage and my half of the booth money, I'd made almost $200.

I lost count of how many customers licked the glass of my booth, staring at my pussy and putting their tongues to the glass as if they were all making out with each other in one big gay orgy of spit and cum. They had to know that other men shot their loads onto the glass, because they themselves did it. And you could see it! By the end of my shift, my glass was covered with cloudy white runnels of ejaculate, with little clean licked spots here and there. *They had to know.*

Were strippers just a conduit for straight men to relate to each other sexually?

"Cold Hard Bitch" — Jet

The next day I got to Eros a little before ten in order to have a few moments to dress before the arcade opened. Stewie was behind the counter, counting piles of ones and fives. His morning face was puffy and old womanish: fiery with blush, orange pancake makeup, and frosted coral lipstick. He looked mean and sneaky, like a pampered old tomcat who sprayed.

"Hi, Stewie," I said. "How are you this morning?"

"Holiday," he sneered.

I didn't think he was going to say anything else, so I slung my backpack onto my shoulder and started to go past the desk toward the windowed hall.

"You did good yesterday," said Stewie, as I passed.

"Huh?"

"You did good. You made us money," he said. I knew it was a compliment, but the way he said the words it sounded like he was adding *you filthy slut* to every declarative statement. I wondered if he would have had more respect for me had I not generated as much income for Eros. Maybe he figured that my shows had to be particularly obscene, because why else would I have made that kind of money?

I'd never understood the snobbery of people in the sex industry who looked askance at the strippers, doms, and models who performed explicit shows. Even other strippers gossip about girls who do "nasty" shows—as if spreading your legs is one thing, but spreading your legs and saying *Fuck me* is another. It seemed to me like the girls doing so-called nasty shows were just doing their jobs better than the girls who were more conflicted about their labor.

"Thank you," I said.

"You're working with Nina and Gigi today," he said.

"Are they back there already?" *Damn.* I'd wanted to work alone again. Rent was coming up and I needed the money. Plus, I hated the thought of competing with two other girls. They were both probably skinny and perfect with brand-new costumes, I thought glumly. My only angle was that I was the new girl, and a lot of customers would see a new girl just for the novelty of seeing a body they hadn't seen at a particular venue before.

I took a deep breath. *Nina and Gigi.* What kind of girls would they be? I couldn't really tell from the names. Sometimes you could tell a lot about a stripper by the name she picked—Ravens were usually dark-haired goths; Diamonds were usually black; clueless women's studies college girls chose names like Jezebel, Salome, or Gaia. But normal names were hard to read.

"Yeah," said Stewie. "Hurry up and get ready. Make us more money today." *You dumb slut, doing your nasty-ass shows.* Stewie's eyes were glassy. I wondered what drugs he could be on to make him so bad-tempered. Maybe nothing—maybe he just hated ladies. But if he *did* hate ladies, why in the world would he choose to work at a peep show? Wouldn't that be like the seventh circle of hell for him, to be around half-naked chicks all day long?

But then again I hated customers, but I wasn't above making money from them.

"Thanks," I said. I went past the desk, down the windowed hall, and to the dressing room door. I heard loud voices, a sudden spray of laughter, then screams.

I knocked loudly. "It's Holiday," I said.

The door was flung open. It seemed that sometimes we'd be locked in, other times not. Over time I came to recognize that there was no underlying pattern or principle to our captivity.

In the doorway, a short, busty woman stood holding on to the doorknob. She didn't move to let me pass. Her legs were very thin, but her dress was tight across her belly. You didn't notice her stomach so much, though, because her tits were so vast. They were like giant saddlebags hanging around her neck. Her cleavage—the line of demarcation between her breasts—was a good ten inches long. She looked like a pretty hen.

Her hair was medium brown and frayed from overprocessing. It looked like it would feel very soft. I guessed her to be somewhere in her mid-thirties, maybe with a kid or two at home to explain the massive tits and her little paunch.

"I'm Holiday," I said again.

"Gigi," she said. "Come on in."

I followed Gigi into the dressing room. Another girl—Nina, I guessed—was putting on fake eyelashes at one of the makeup counters. With only one set of eyelashes on she had a charming, fiendish look, like Malcolm McDowell in *A Clockwork Orange*. Cosmetics were strewn across the table, most opened and some spilled or smeared. *So much for my clean table,* I thought.

Nina was topless. Her breasts were tiny—just nipples, hard buttons on the field of her chest. Her shoulders were broad and angular, leading down to a fine, strong back. She was tall, with long slender legs, and her hair was cut into a severe bob and dyed black. She wore bright red lipstick. I wondered if it was the same Wet 'n' Wild shade I wore.

"Hello," I said. "I'm Holiday." Instantly I felt like an idiot—how many times was I going to introduce myself? She had to have heard me at the door, saying my name to Gigi.

"*A cheap holiday, in other people's misery!*" Nina sang, doing a passable Johnny Rotten. She and Gigi howled. She continued to sing as I put my backpack down on the other makeup table.

I was wary—who were these girls? Who might be an ally? Could they possibly be friendly? Were they going to be cutthroat, forming an alliance with each other to force me out? I watched them covertly, greedily snatching as much information as I could from their facial expressions and body language.

Gigi seemed relaxed, but Nina was freaking me out—she was definitely the looser cannon of the two, the alpha dog. I hoped we wouldn't have to get down to it, sparring over pack leadership in some kind of ridiculous stripper rumble. I just wanted to work—I didn't want to be stolen from, beat up, or sabotaged! I wasn't there to make friends, or infringe on anyone else's business. We could all ply our trades without stepping on one another's toes—that was, if Nina didn't feel the need to establish supremacy by taking a stand against the unwelcome intrusion of a new girl. Maybe she was just blowing off steam and if I let her amuse herself, she'd get bored and turn her focus elsewhere. I just hoped I wasn't about to be jumped.

"Did you pick your name from the Madonna song?" asked Nina. Without waiting for my answer, she started singing Madonna's "Holiday." Gigi giggled. Nina howled, pounding the makeup counter with the flat of her palm in exaggerated, theatrical amusement.

"I picked it off the Holiday Inn down the street," I said quietly. Both girls stopped laughing and stared at me.

I stared back.

Nina screamed.

"Fuck yeah!" she shrieked. "Holiday fucking *Inn!*"

It was chaos. I was getting a headache from all the yelling, but at least Nina was laughing *with* me, instead of caterwauling songs *at* me. And Gigi had turned toward the mirror, dismissing us both in order to apply liquid eyeliner, removing some of Nina's motivation to perform. It was past ten, so I dressed quickly, getting into the same costume I'd worn the day before. Miraculously, Nina's maniacal giggling subsided. Scowling into the mirror in focused concentration, she applied her other set of false eyelashes. I began to relax in tiny increments, ratcheting my anxiety down notch by notch as the three of us finished dressing and getting made up.

When I pulled out my blond wig, Gigi asked, "You don't use your own hair?"

"Nah," I said. I shook the wig out, and put it on over my wig cap. "It's more insane this way."

"They like blondes," said Gigi, speculatively.

"I aim to please," I said.

Finishing her eyelashes, Nina pirouetted around the dressing room, singing to herself. She was a tornado, a force of nature. Everything in the room was subject to her: She picked up makeup and tossed it down, peed without closing the door to the tiny bathroom, seized pieces of my costume, held them up, and dropped them, ruffled Gigi's feathery hair, and provided a running, sung commentary. Her volume in the small room made her inescapable. Her long legs were everywhere. Her laugh rang out like shots fired.

I felt tired just watching her.

Nina was crazy. I mean, she was crazy in the way crazy people are crazy—she was *manic*. She burned all the energy in the room, turning oxygen into the fire that fueled her constant noise and motion. I felt like I moved in slow motion next to her. I was cold and sluggish, and she was white-hot and crackling.

The stage lights lowered, then brightened again.

"Stage," said Gigi. "You want it?"

"No," I said. I wanted to be polite, since they'd gotten to work first. "Go ahead."

"*I want it!*" screamed Nina. She dashed up the steps to the stage.

"Have you worked here before?" Gigi asked me. She was using a small, slotted brush to smooth her hair down. Her face was round and kind. She looked like one of my mom's friends. Maybe having kids made you so tired, you became gentle.

"Yeah," I said. "Yesterday."

"You know about the tip slots in the booths?"

Tip slots in the booths? There were *no tip slots in the booths!* At least I didn't think there were.

"No," I said. "Are you talking about the tip slots onstage?"

"Nuh-uh," Gigi said. "Come here." She put her brush down and led me over to one of the boxes.

She kicked off her shoes and crawled into the cubicle, hoisting herself up with a slight grunt. *Strong little chicken wings,* I thought, *to lift up all that bosom.*

"Hand me a magazine," she said, pointing toward an old, ragged pile of out-of-date periodicals that lived on top of the mini fridge. Most of them lacked covers, and some were swollen and buckled with water damage. I'd read most of them the day before, in between customers, though some smelled like pee and I didn't touch those. It seemed like everything at Eros smelled like urine. I hoped the smell wasn't getting into my wig hair.

I grabbed the first magazine that wasn't too battered and handed it to Gigi.

"Okay," she said. "Here's how you get your tips from booth shows."

She ripped out a subscription postcard from the magazine. Then she used the card to inch around the edge of the window until she found a minute gap between the glass and the frame. Then she pushed the postcard through the gap. I saw it sticking out on the customers' side of the glass. *Holy shit! Houston, we have contact!* It was weird to think of us being able to insert things into the customers' side of the booth. It looked like an optical illusion, like she was pushing the postcard through a solid wall.

She wiggled the card. "Tell them to put their tips through the gap. Shake the card so they'll see where."

I was astonished. "They'll *do* that?"

"Yeah," she said. "The ones who've been here before, they know to do that automatically. The new guys, you have to train them. Just wiggle the card and tell them to put your money through the window."

Fuck! I had given up so much money—*my tip money*—to Eros yesterday. I'd gone home with $200, but if I'd known to make them put money through the gap, I could have made over a hundred dollars more.

"Thank you," I said. "Really. That's awesome."

"Yeah," said Gigi. "Here, you can keep this card. I've got my own in my locker."

"Thanks," I said.

"Don't tell Baby Jane, up front," Gigi said.

Her admonition was unnecessary. I couldn't imagine telling Stewie anything, let alone informing him about a dodge to keep all my tip money instead of splitting it with the house. "Of course not," I said.

"Hey! I need more money!"

The scream came from onstage. Nina.

"Give me more fucking money, you dick!" I heard the slap of angry hands against glass.

"Well, fuck you then, bitch," Nina said, strutting back into the dressing room from the stage.

"Is he gone?" I asked.

"No. But he stopped tipping, so he can fucking stand there by himself. I'm not working for free." She tossed handfuls of ones onto her makeup table.

I hadn't realized you could walk off like that. But now that I knew you could, I planned to remember that and use it as leverage. *Punishment.*

I really liked Gigi and Nina. Nina scared the hell out of me, but that was okay.

I had a feeling she terrorized the customers much more.

"Little Sister"—
Queens of the Stone Age

It turned out Nina and Gigi had been working at Eros for over five years. They didn't share housing, but they scheduled every shift together so they could work as a team. I watched them share costumes, makeup, gum, and a cell phone indiscriminately.

At one o'clock Gigi unpacked lunch for both of them, laying it out on the table and folding paper towels from the bathroom into big triangles, like napkins. They ate together, quickly and efficiently. When they were done, Nina washed out the Tupperware in the bathroom sink and put it back in Gigi's carryall, then they briefly discussed what they wanted to have for lunch the next day. They appeared to be effectively married to each other, conducting the small business of their lives in cheerful conjunction.

I'd noticed both of them putting the cash they made into one zippered makeup bag on the table claimed by Nina's cosmetics. When Gigi saw me looking, she said, "We split our take."

I didn't get it. "With the house?"

"No," she said. "With each other. We put all our money in there, and at the end of the shift, we split it. That way we don't have to go head-to-head."

It made perfect sense. The terrible thing about working with friends was that if you got the customer's money, you felt bad because you got picked over your friend—but if your friend got his money, you felt bad because you didn't get picked. There was no way to win—unless you refused to compete with your comrades and worked out a way so that everyone profited together. When either Nina or Gigi had a bad day at work—and everyone did eventually; no one was immune—it didn't matter, because there was no jealousy or resentment or pity between them. They took care of each other.

Nina taught me how to get exorbitant tips onstage. She'd approach the tip slot and instead of requesting or demanding money to dance, she'd whisper, "Listen: A straight fuck is a hundred and twenty dollars. Put it through here."

If the customers attempted to ask questions or clarify, Nina would silence them immediately. "Do you want to get us busted? Put it through, and I'll meet you in the back booth, *ése.*" Any further objections on the part of the customer would be viciously hushed.

If the customer was intrigued and hopeful—but vacillating—she'd hiss, "Do you have a condom?"

I think the customers believed that such a pragmatic concern on Nina's part signified the probability of the act of prostitution actually occurring. It was like saying, *Hang on a minute, I have to take my tampon out.* The artlessness of the question sold the fantasy.

Of course, a lot of customers wouldn't bite, even when asked if they had prophylactics. But every now and again Nina came back into the dressing room with a roll of bills in her hand, crowing in triumph. A little bit after that we'd hear angry pounding and banging from the back booth, which we ignored. Eventually Stewie would come and bounce the customer, who would be yelling about having been ripped off by a dancer.

But what could the angry customer do? He couldn't call the police and accuse anyone of anything, because then he'd have to admit to soliciting acts of prostitution. He'd be just as guilty as Nina. And Nina could just claim he'd tipped her, then gotten mad that she'd refused to meet him later. It was diabolical.

I got skilled at working my magazine subscription postcard through the unsealed molding around my booth's window. Each box had a gap that had been painstakingly enlarged by a series of canny occupants—the locations passed along from stripper to stripper—so that we could keep all of the money we negotiated. I learned to tell the customers to put $10 into the bill collector, which raised the curtain and started the show. Anything else I demanded went through the gap in the window.

I brought toys, which I set on paper towels in the hallway window of my cubicle. When customers strolled by I smacked the glass and pointed to the biggest plastic dick I had. Sometimes I licked it. You had to be really careful about licking toys, though, because if Seattle Vice caught us penetrating ourselves—even orally—we could have gotten busted for prostitution. It was on the books. So we were careful to put our tongues way out in order to lick the toys—we never inserted them *into* our mouths. Of course, once a customer was in the booth frantically jerking his cock you could be pretty sure he wasn't Vice, and you could shove your toys into whatever orifice the customer paid enough money to watch you penetrate.

Most of the customers wanted to come on our faces. I learned to put my face as close to the window as possible, lying on my back and opening my mouth. When I saw the white splashes on the glass my job was done. It was relaxing to lie down. I could fit on the floor of the box if I bent my knees. My coat felt soft, like a wool blanket.

The stranglers were mildly upsetting at first, until I got used to them. They liked the fantasy of choking us: They put their hands up to the glass and we presented our necks, as if for throttling. Sometimes they paid us to choke ourselves: They liked watching us turn red and make gasping noises. The glass made me courageous. I would have been much more reluctant to perform that kind of show had I not been safely enclosed in my plastic cube. I was surprised at how many normal-seeming men got hard at the thought of killing women slowly, through strangulation. Maybe I wasn't surprised at how much they wanted to fantasize about choking us, but more by their lack of shame in asking us to perform such a grisly act to their specifications.

But honestly, all they had to do was pay us. We weren't there to suggest counseling. And doing the fetishy stuff was less boring than just plunging my guts, front and back, with a series of plastic cocks. Fetish shows paid more and allowed for a measure of creativity as well. Sure, the choking shows were creepy, but so was calling a customer "Daddy" and wearing a Catholic schoolgirl outfit, or finger-fucking my own asshole—services I also provided. Fetish shows were like "nasty" shows: The only girls not doing them were the ones who were morally conflicted about the nature of their work in the first place, and who desperately needed to claim some kind of moral high ground.

I worked with Nina and Gigi a lot, but I also met a slew of other girls who worked at Eros. Nobody worked full-time— you really couldn't. Even thirty hours a week in a plastic box was physically exhausting. Most of us worked fifteen to twenty hours a week to prevent burnout, making enough to pay our bills without becoming mentally unhinged by the claustrophobia and the constant, belligerent haggling.

I'd thought Nina was nuts, but she was nothing compared to some of my coworkers. I was beginning to understand—to really deeply *comprehend*—what Crystal had said about the peeps being like jail. We were all crazier than shithouse rats. We were boxed up and in each other's way constantly, trapped in a single-sex environment, and forced to deal with other women's bodies intimately. We had to hustle to get the customers to take shows, and once we got them in their stalls, we had to hustle them even harder to get their money. Many girls smoked and there was no ventilation or fresh air of any kind—just the pee smell. Nearly everyone drank or used drugs to combat the monumental boredom of a slow day, though I preferred not to. I figured I was probably sucking up enough secondhand cigarette and weed smoke as it was.

There were fights, grudges, alliances, epic vendettas, and most of all, gossip. Revenge was fast and merciless. A favored method of guerrilla assault was pouring undiluted bleach on a girl's costume kit while she was in her box performing, or cutting the ankle straps on her shoes. There were fistfights, screaming verbal altercations, and bouts of deliberate intimidation. I learned not to smile, to stake out my space and jealously guard it.

Holding my ground at Eros—getting the box I preferred, keeping my belongings safe, and not getting my money stolen— required a unique combination of hostility and imagination. When a big Jamaican girl working under the name Queenie tried to tell me I'd done a show for one of her regular customers— and that I owed her half the money from the show because of that—I told her to suck my fucking dick. I didn't want to fight but if I gave her what she wanted even once, I knew I'd be subject to her will forever. Later, for payback, I told all her regular customers she had rampant genital herpes, halving her income for weeks.

There was absolutely no regulation of any kind, and no help from Stewie. He liked it when we fought, or when a girl went home robbed and crying. He was like a vampire, battening on the waves of our turbulence. He only looked depressed when we were making money, mellowed out, and temporarily in truce.

I thought that if Stewie were heterosexual, he'd probably be a strangler.

Behind the cum-streaked glass, I was safe and unreachable. I felt myself growing a hard exoskeleton, becoming armored. I liked my tough shell.

"Cherry Pie" — Warrant

Every bit of money I could steal from the customers at Eros, I stole. I used Nina's condom trick whenever I thought the customer seemed naive or distracted enough to go for it, and I made every single booth customer flatten out his bills and slip them through the tiny crack in the molding of the window. Eros Galaxy was making about $40 per day from me in booth fees, while I was going home with hundreds of wadded-up bills stuffed into my costume kit.

"How come you made so much money on your first shift and now you're doing so *shitty*, Holiday?" Stewie asked one night while he was cashing me out. He enjoyed counting the bills slowly when we had cabs outside, knowing that most taxi drivers ran their meters while they waited for working girls. His voice was a slow drawl, exaggeratedly enervated. He sounded like a big, mean Blanche DuBois in an all-transvestite production of *A Streetcar Named Desire*.

"I don't know, Stewie—beginner's luck?" I said, shrugging. "But that was then—I'm not the new girl anymore." I looked down the stairway: Sure enough, my cab sat in the loading zone in front of the building. I imagined the meter ticking away, counting off dollars in twenty-cent increments. I forced myself to relax— what would the fare be, an extra $5? I'd made over $400 that night. Stewie's sadism was only annoying because it was so small and constantly expressed—like a radio station turned down but always on, or someone kicking the back of your seat all through a movie. It seemed like he never got tired of making our lives slightly more unpleasant.

"You're still kind of new," Stewie whined. "Lots of *clients* haven't seen you." Stewie yelled at us constantly for referring to the cum-licking habitués of Eros as *customers*. Maybe he thought calling them *clients* lent us an air of polish and class, as if they were wealthy businessmen and we were investment bankers being paid to manage their portfolios instead of strangling ourselves and finger-fucking our own assholes. Or maybe he just liked to tell us what to do, and the whole client/customer thing was merely a convenient ruse. His mean baby-doll eyes glittered as he counted and recounted my money, extravagantly snapping the bills like a casino dealer. I half expected him to clap briskly and turn his palms up—*nothing up my sleeve*—for imaginary casino security cams behind black glass globes in the ceiling.

I wondered if anyone loved Stewie. Anyone at all. Or if anyone ever had. There were rumors that Stewie lived with a boyfriend, but nobody had ever seen the boyfriend and Stewie had never been observed taking a personal phone call of any sort. I suspected that if Stewie did in fact have a boyfriend, he probably lived in a hole down in Stewie's basement, rubbing lotion on his skin and fearing the hose.

"Yeah, but I've lost that new-car smell," I said. "And besides, it's been slow."

True: It was slow—for Eros. Only a few dozen customers had come in that night. Of course, I'd extorted nearly every single one of them and made more money punishing them than Stewie made in a week.

I was tired: My feet hurt, and the big muscles on my thighs felt like they'd been punched. They were stretched out and achy from my platform stiletto shoes, which forced my heels up high and made the muscles along the front of my legs pull taut. I liked the pain; I was used to it. It meant I was working, and making money.

A customer came up the stairway and stopped dead in his tracks, at the far end of the counter. He stared from me to the money on the counter, then back at me again.

"Holiday . . . ?" he said. "Is that you?"

"Yeah," I snapped. "Just going home, as soon as the floor man finishes *fondling* my money."

I made sure to say *floor man* instead of *manager*. Stewie hated that, I knew. I'd heard him tell a new girl he was the *shift supervisor* once, and I'd been laughing at that ever since. The peeps was no place for delusions of grandeur. Ultimately, he was just a sad old queer who worked at the peep show because nobody would hassle him about his makeup or his queenish ways, and because nobody else wanted to mop up jizz for forty hours a week. Calling Stewie a *shift supervisor* was like calling me a Las Vegas–style showgirl: Neither title had anything to do with men paying by the minute to lick up each other's ejaculate.

Stewie glared at me, pursing his little pink-frosted anus-mouth.

"You look different," the customer said. "Did you dye your hair?" He gazed at me, horrified.

All of a sudden I saw what he was seeing: his fantasy girl, but torn down from her pedestal, smashed in the face a few times, and kicked around the block.

I was *not* the Holiday he'd jerked off to. I wasn't even a Las Vegas–style showgirl.

I stared at myself in the mirror behind the counter.

The wig cap had left my hair wet with sweat, clumped and frizzy. My real hair was brown—not platinum blond—and it was twisted into two sloppy braids, instead of hanging loose and silky down to my shoulders.

My eye makeup had somehow slid from mostly *over* my eyes to mostly *under* them. All the black liner and mascara I wore was caked into the fine lines under my eyes, some of it crumbling down onto my cheeks. My face was flushed and greasy. I'd wiped most of my lipstick off with the back of my hand, but some of it was still smeared around my mouth, giving me a rabid, bloodthirsty look. The hand I'd wiped my mouth with was stained murderously red, Lady Macbethishly.

Instead of long nylons and a tiny slip, I wore sweatpants and a Slayer shirt that still had mustard on it from the sandwich I'd had for dinner the night before. Holiday didn't eat (nor did Las Vegas showgirls, as far as I knew), but I was usually ravenous after a day of work. We weren't allowed to leave during our shifts, so if you didn't bring food, you had to wait to eat until you got off. Most nights I stopped at the all-night grocery store on my way home.

Unlike ballerinas, strippers tend to gorge like lumberjacks: We move and dance and sweat and run and assume tricky positions all day long, so when we feed, we do so with a rather alarming amount of gusto. I'd learned to pick out fellow dancers in Seattle's handful of twenty-four-hour restaurants: They were the sort-of-cute ones in loose boy-clothes and no makeup, gobbling down plates of heavy food late at night. We tipped well and liked to be left alone with our food.

I realized my customer hadn't left. He was still standing in front of the counter, frozen. He, Stewie, and I made a tableau, like the central triangle grouping in da Vinci's *Last Supper*. Stewie was Jesus. I was Judas.

It figured.

I chipped at the yellow mustard crust on my shirt with my thumbnail. It smelled vinegary and good. I was starving.

I had no inclination to explain to the customer that Holiday was not, in fact, real. That she was smoke and mirrors and voodoo and glamour. That there *was* no Holiday, and never *would* be. That *no* woman was Holiday—no woman could be. Like Barbie with her impossible anatomy, a real Holiday could not exist. She was made of cheap satin and cosmetic wax and doll hair and vanilla-scented body spray, and that was that.

I realized I stank. I'd put on makeup, sweated it off, put on more, and sweated through that again. All day long. Now I looked demented, and the foundation and powder caked on my skin made me look like I'd been spackled with wet Bisquick.

As the customer stared at me, in the full light of the arcade lobby, with no sperm-frosted glass between us to soften my lines and blur me into a more perfect fantasy—with me about seven inches shorter in flat shoes instead of heels; with my big tits flattened against my chest by my minimizer bra instead of fluffed up and presented on a bed of pressed foam and cheap lace—his shock and disappointment were palpable. "Oh," he said, softly. "Well, you look—different."

I couldn't argue with that.

Suddenly I remembered him. He'd stood in my booth about a week ago, legs spread, jerking his perfectly average cock. The only thing notable about him was that he chose to orgasm into a wad of tissues, instead of onto the glass or floor, like most of the other *clients*. And after he was done, he'd asked me if I had a boyfriend. When I said no, he'd invited me out to dinner. Our encounter had been almost like a date, albeit a really bad and backward one.

Stewie finished counting my money, handed me my cut—a superfluous $35, considering how much I'd actually made—and I walked past the customer and down to my cab. His eyes looked wounded.

The message in them was clear: *You tricked me.*

His pain was so sincere that I felt bad, as if I'd just told a three-year-old that Santa Claus was actually just his mom and dad.

He'd really *believed* in Holiday.

Chapter 4
Fetish and Domination

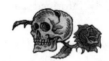

"Hell"—
Squirrel Nut Zippers

My first client of the day at Butterscotch's was Luis the Mexican Ass Man, who promptly informed me that he wanted to eat my shit.

That was a new angle for him—I'd been seeing him for months, and usually he just wanted to converse about licking and fucking my asshole, the salacious discussion of which I gladly provided for the cost of a fetish show. The shit-talk didn't surprise me though, because Luis was obsessed with butts: mine, his own, and everyone else's. Shit seemed to be a reasonable extension of his obsession.

Luis's own ass was seemingly endlessly capacious. It stretched out willingly for whatever he put into it, including all five of his own fingers past the saddle of his knuckles. The inside of his ass was pink and looked like segmented rubber tubing.

Once Luis brought a can of Country Scent Lysol to his session, which he then inserted all the way into his own rectum, bottom end first. He asked me if it turned me on to watch him fuck his own ass with the Lysol. I told him that of course it did—that all women secretly wanted their men to fuck themselves with aerosol cans, and that I felt very lucky to be living out that particular fantasy in his pleasant company. After his session he made sure to take the Lysol with him, tucking it into his coat pocket carefully. I devoutly hoped he wasn't taking it home to clean and disinfect surfaces.

It was hard to get money out of Luis, so I had to resort to all kinds of tricks to get him to tip me. In this particular session I ended up briefly excusing myself and using my brown eyeliner pencil to draw shit streaks into the crotch of an old thong I had in my costume kit. When I came back with the "dirty" panties in my hand, Luis was delighted. I sold them to him for $60, then watched as he sniffed and chewed the eyeliner right out of the fabric.

"Emma, I eat your *sheet,*" he kept saying.

"*Sí,* Luis, you're eating my shit," I confirmed. I wondered if he was concerned about the fact that my shit tasted of nothing more than cosmetic-grade pigment and wax.

"Flippin' tha Bird" — Ruby

Summer slipped into autumn.

I worked mostly with Viva and Lenore, though there were a few other girls who worked at Butterscotch's regularly. None of us were full-time. Why bother, when you made enough to live nicely on working three or four short shifts a week?

I was a little surprised to find that I had become if not an old girl myself, at least someone who was accepted by the old guard. Crystal, Lenore, and Viva formed the backbone of Butterscotch's. When they complained to me about the stupidity, vanity, or duplicity of new hires, I realized both that they considered me an experienced, reliable worker and that they had turned from coworkers into friends. I particularly looked forward to my shifts with Viva. I never tired of watching her put on her complicated mask of makeup, using little foam swabs to daub on eye shadow from her half dozen identical pots of color.

I learned to dread new girls along with the others because of the way customers would flock to them and attempt to get them to perform illegal acts, like touching or flashing. A lot of the new girls were naive enough to do those things, and were effortlessly manipulated by the customers. Even worse, they'd do it for no extra money. They'd do it just because the customers told them to. That was one of the first things we'd tell new hires at Butterscotch's: *Don't let the customers tell you what to do,* ever.

A new girl got fired for blowing on a customer's balls. Another one got fired for rubbing a customer's cock with her bare feet. She cried and protested that she hadn't touched him. "Touching's with hands!" she wept. Crystal put her costumes in a plastic grocery sack and made her leave halfway through her shift.

There was little room for sympathy, and no excuse for mistakes—if one girl got busted for prostitution, we'd all get taken in. Seattle Vice visited us constantly, pretending to be legitimate, horny customers, trying to trick us into nudity or touch. We had to police each other to keep ourselves safe. The showrooms had cameras behind the wall mirrors, and Crystal had to watch the tapes of everyone's sessions to make sure each model kept visible space between herself and her customer. If we performed our jobs as trained, there was no problem.

The fact that the customers masturbated was a legal gray area: If we, the models, complained to the police that a client had exposed himself and masturbated, the charge would be public lewdness and the client risked ticketing. We didn't complain, though, so technically there was no crime happening. It was like that old zen koan, *If a tree falls in the forest and there's no one to hear it, does it make a sound?* The answer—at least at Butterscotch's—was, *No, it doesn't make a sound.*

I was late for a shift at Butterscotch's. "Stripper time" was a very real phenomenon—most working girls chronically ran fifteen to thirty minutes behind schedule. "I'm on stripper time," we'd say, shrugging, in lieu of apology for showing up late to our shifts—but I was an hour late to my shift, and that was pushing it. I hated having to get dressed and made up under pressure, but I'd been making a new dance tape for work and had lost track of time. Also, I was working with Viva, who tended to be less tolerant of stripper time than Lenore, who gleefully invoked that excuse herself nearly every shift.

I rushed through the front door and down the hall. When I got to the dressing room, Viva was getting dressed in her black PVC for a domination session. She looked like a shiny black bug, beautiful and frightening, with her drawn-on eyebrows arching like antennae. I imagined myself on my knees, licking her knee-high boots. They looked like they'd taste of licorice until she kicked me in the face, and then I'd only taste blood.

She was wearing a blond wig with her dreads tucked up underneath. I could see sweat at her hairline, from hurrying her dressing. *"Fuck,"* she growled. "You're actually here. Good, because I sold this dude a two-mistress show."

"Seriously?" I said. "Okay, give me a minute." It figured—on the day I was over an hour late, I'd come in and have to do a complicated two-girl dom session right away. I hastily applied black eye pencil and mascara, adding a little extra in an attempt to look suitably fiendish.

Viva said, "He's easy. I've seen him a million times before." She worked an opera-length glove over her hand, then rolled it up one skinny arm. "His name is Chris, but he likes to be called Christine. He wants to be a little slut. Just tell him he's a nasty little bitch, and make him jack off. He wants two girls to humiliate him."

I put on lipstick and blotted my mouth with toilet paper from a roll we kept on the makeup counter. "Can I follow your lead?" I asked.

"Yeah," Viva said. "But seriously, he's just happy to be here. He's totally simple. He's not a tipper, though, so don't knock yourself out."

I dressed rapidly. I wore my black evening dress with the silver sparkles, a satin corset laced tightly over the dress, and my long black gloves. I felt like I spent half my life in the kind of clothes most women only wore on Halloween.

We entered the dungeon together. I'd been in there for sessions many times before, but I'd never gotten used to how small and cramped the space seemed. The human-size cage, the cross, and the little tables with baskets of rope and clamps were crowded together in a room just slightly bigger than one of the veal pens. To add to the claustrophobia, the walls were hung with equipment—floggers, paddles, belts, handcuffs, and single-tailed whips. I stood by the cross, and Viva took up a position near the wall of implements.

The customer, Chris—*Christine,* I reminded myself—was in the cage, dressed in frilly white underwear. He already stank of sweat. As we entered, he peered at us through the bars pathetically, luxuriating in the sensual fear he'd purchased with his credit card. "Oh, Mistresses . . ." he whispered happily.

Viva took a riding crop off one of the hooks on the wall. She slapped it against the bars of the cage. The sound of the leather against the metal was incredibly loud and terrifying, and Chris shrank back against the back bars of the cage. Each slap sounded like if it hit flesh—instead of the bars of the cage—it would sting like a snakebite. I jumped at each resounding *thwack* and tried to keep my face neutral.

"Shut the fuck up, bitch," she said. "Did I tell you to talk?"

Chris was silent in his cage.

"Crawl out," Viva said.

Chris cautiously opened the door to the cage, which was unlocked. He crawled out on his hands and knees, then knelt in front of Viva.

"I want you to meet Mistress Emma," she said. "She's here to help with your slut training."

Chris looked at me. I stared into his face for a long moment, keeping him waiting.

"Keep your eyes down, whore," I finally said, quietly.

Immediately Chris looked down, his face coloring in embarrassment and delight.

I noticed his cock, hard against the fabric of his white frilly panties. They had ruffles on the bottom, like the panties some parents imposed on their little girls. I wondered where in the world you bought man-size little-girl panties. Online, maybe? Would everyone know you were buying them for yourself, or could you pretend you were buying them for your freakishly large toddler? I wondered if he wore his little-girl fetish panties under his regular clothes all the time. They even had little strawberries on them.

Viva selected a few clamps from a basket on the table. "Why don't you clamp her slutty little nipples, Mistress Emma?" she asked me. "That ought to teach her a lesson."

She handed me the clamps. I put them on the customer's nipples. At first I didn't pinch enough skin, and they fell off. Then I opened them wider and shoved them on, savagely, getting big folds of skin between the serrated jaws of the clamps. Chris moaned. His nipples already looked bruised and raw, as tender as rare steak tips.

"That's what you get, you dirty little slut," I said. "Does it hurt?"

"Yes, ma'am," Chris whispered. He hung his head exultantly.

Viva tied Chris's hands behind his back, just above the ruffles of his panties. Her corset creaked as she bent to tie the knots.

"Guess what, Christine?" said Viva. "This is what happens to nasty little bitches who can't keep their legs closed." She slapped him lightly in the face.

And again.

And again. Back and forth. It was hypnotizing.

As I watched Viva hit our customer in the face, I considered my options. I didn't want to touch him—his back was slick with sweat. I could see little curls of his armpit hair soaked in perspiration and glued against his skin. He was panting—big, open-mouthed gulps of air. He gasped as Viva's hand cracked across his face again, the sound of the slap unbearably loud in such close quarters.

I took a deep breath.

"You wet-pussied little whore," I said. "You sloppy-gashed piece of slut *fuck*. You think you're something precious, don't you. All dressed up in your stupid little white panties. But all of us know the kind of girl you really are, you cock-sucking, cunt-spreading little *harlot.*"

Viva stared past me. I'd never seen her look surprised before. None of us moved.

Harlot? I thought.

"Do you think you're special, you *bitch?* You daddy's girl? You nasty piece of cock-loving trash?"

It was like I was possessed. Bad and profane words kept falling out of my mouth, connected by innocent little words like *you* and *and.* I felt sorry for the good words that had to hook all the hideous ones together. It didn't seem fair. My hair felt tight on my scalp, like I was bristling or being electrocuted. I couldn't stop.

"You . . . you cheap, lazy, ass-fucked *strumpet.* You make me *sick.* You cum-gobbling, gang-banged, loose-pussied whore."

Viva slapped Chris in the face again. Hard. It was like punctuation.

With a mucusy gasp that sounded like tearing paper, Chris came in his panties. We didn't see it happen, but we saw his hips buck twice, hard, and the spreading wet stain in the crotch of his drawers was unmistakable.

So was the smell. I needed air. The room seemed unendurably hot. I couldn't breathe—had I laced my corset tighter than usual? Wearing it over my gown had been a mistake. Viva, on the other hand, looked cool and comfortable in her corset and thong panties. I sighed, feeling like a rank amateur.

Viva untied our customer's hands and handed him one of the ubiquitous washcloths that were piled throughout Butterscotch's. "Clean yourself up," she said. She spread a towel on the floor. "When you're done, put your dirty washcloth here. *Not* on the carpet, or the table."

We walked out of the dungeon together and stood leaning against the wall, allowing Chris to clean himself up and dress in privacy. We could hear him getting dressed through the door of the dungeon—it sounded like he had a lot of loose change in his pockets. I wondered if he'd brought underwear to change into, or if he was just planning on wearing the ruffly, cummy toddler panties home.

I didn't feel any sense of power, even though we'd been paid to dominate Chris and treat him as our inferior. Mostly, I just felt confused—was our session really over? Was that really all he'd wanted—a bunch of arcane insults, and a little face-slapping? I honestly didn't know why they even came to see us. It seemed like such a sad and embarrassing way to spend money, paying strangers to treat you with contempt.

Viva said, "Oh my god, did you really call him a strumpet?"

"Yes."

"That's pretty fucking funny. Isn't that from the Bible?"

I looked at her, but I wasn't sure if she was smiling. Possibly— her lips were twisted up at the corners. She was staring at the wall.

"Peek-a-Boo"—
Siouxsie and the Banshees

The first time I peed for the camera, I drank liters of water and soda pop and coffee in preparation, though I'd refused beer because I didn't want to appear tipsily bloated and red-faced on film. The photographer gave me a handful of diuretics, which I swallowed with several bottles of water. The shoot entailed me peeing into a kiddie pool, a cat box, and various glasses and bowls. It lasted six hours and paid $150 per hour. At one point, while attempting to relax so I could release my bladder into an oversize brandy snifter, I'd farted—loudly—but that was no more embarrassing than squatting and urinating into a boxful of Tidy Cats, so I just laughed and kept peeing on cue.

I took every modeling job I could, not because I needed the money but because I couldn't stand to turn money down—and because the more I worked, the more work I was offered. I scheduled shoots weeks in advance, weaving them around my shifts at Butterscotch's and Eros Galaxy.

It was like being the school slut: Once word gets around that you'll spread your legs, everyone stands in line to fuck you. I didn't care about being respected, or about appearing not to have standards. The money was what was important. At the end of the day, did it matter if I did one photo shoot or a hundred? Or if I only did closed-legged "art" modeling or pissed into glasses and fucked myself with hair-conditioner-covered toys for hardcore shoots? Either way, my pussy was still plastered all over the Internet.

It occurred to me once during a video shoot, while I was sucking on a large black dildo, that my definition of *embarrassing* had been turned way, way down. It was as if my sense of shame had been injected with Botox: I knew it was there, but I couldn't feel it at all.

I was pretty much done with Butterscotch's—it just wasn't worth showing up for shifts and prancing around in lingerie when I could make more doing hardcore modeling. I gave two weeks' notice to Crystal on my next shift, and when my two weeks were up, the other girls bought me a cake from a local gourmet bakery to celebrate my "moving on." *Moving on* sounded like *passing on* to me, like I was dead but not forgotten. The cake was rum-chocolate—bittersweet with dark chocolate ganache and a raspberry preserve filling. We ate it from paper plates in the dressing room as we listened for the door.

Chapter 5
Holy Hand Jobs

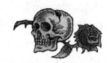

"Cemetery Gates" — Pantera

I'd never thought filth and shocking sexual perversion would become routine, but they had. Playing Let's Pretend with a variety of men with their dicks in their hands and being rewarded by gouts of cum on the other side of the glass wasn't a novelty anymore—it was just my life, and it had become stultifying.

More concretely, Stewie had hired a little blond stripper named Taya who pretended to female ejaculate for customers, but because what she was actually doing was peeing on the plastic floor of her box, the whole place smelled pissier than usual. I was sick of coming in ten minutes early to every shift to clean dried stripper pee off my performance space. The whole place smelled like a nursing home, and was about as depressing.

Furthermore, the sad, cutout Christmas decorations taped to the walls of the arcade seemed designed to inspire holiday suicide. The customers ignored them, but I felt like the cartoon Santas and reindeer on the wall threw the pee smell and all the unholy human degeneracy that occurred on both sides of the curtained glass into sharp relief. I figured Stewie had put the decorations up to torture us, in a mean-spirited attempt to make our jobs uncomfortable and joyless during the holiday season. After all, he didn't have to stare at the Christmas stuff all day long—he was behind the front desk, watching his portable TV and making change for the customers, so they could pay us dollar by dollar and maybe save themselves a few bucks by coming as fast as they could. The only people affected by the decorations were us, the strippers. They were directly across the hall from our boxes, taped at eye level. I had to think that was on purpose.

Stewie accepted my leave of absence with a shrug. "I'll just schedule Taya for your shifts, Holiday," he said pettishly. "The customers like her better anyway, because she doesn't have your *weight problem.*"

"I thought they liked her better because she pees all over herself for twenty bucks, Stewie," I said. In spite of his meanness, I felt merry. I wasn't sure if it was the spirit of the season, or if it was just the thought of leaving Eros Galaxy to simmer in its own urine-scented depravity.

We stared at each other in mutual animosity for a moment. Stewie's cheeks flushed red under his baby-doll makeup.

Finally, he said, "Just go. Make sure you get all your shit out of your locker."

I took a few weeks off, stayed home, and watched lots of TV. It was delightful not to have to see any penises at all. To celebrate, I grew out my pubic hair. My sense of bodily privacy was a heady thing, even though the new hair made my pussy itch abominably.

Another peep show girl had told me about a workplace that intrigued me. It was a massage place, meaning I'd have to actually touch penises instead of just talking to them through glass—but after so many years, touching seemed like a natural gradation of my work, and not something to be overly distressed about. True, touching was prostitution—a fully illegal act on the books, unlike the semi-illegal stuff I was already doing, like penetrating myself in my box at Eros Galaxy and rubbing my own pussy through my panties at Butterscotch's. If I were to mistakenly touch a cop—or even *agree* to touch a cop—I'd be arrested and ticketed. I'd have a prostitution strike on my record, and my record would be available to the public. It gave me pause.

But what ultimately proved attractive about the place was the idea of not having to constantly *pretend*. If I offered touch, I could simply perform the service I was offering, with no exhausting psychosexual role-playing. Men would come in, I'd jerk them off, and they'd leave. I could be a dairymaid, just milking away in silence, keeping my thoughts to myself. I wouldn't have to entertain or enchant or titillate the cows, or pretend to milk myself, or try to convince them that the milking felt just as good for me as it did for them. Paradoxically, by offering more service, I would actually be providing less interaction.

Plus, I had to admit I was curious. Would I feel any different going from live modeling and dancing to actual hands-on service? Maybe it would feel good to be so honest and pragmatic.

I had to admit something to myself after more than half a decade spent rolling in filth for pay: When I came across something in the adult industry that seemed dangerous or scary, there was only a small part of me that said *Avoid, avoid!* Everything else in me needed to leap into the fray. It's like I couldn't *not* investigate once I knew something bad was out there that I hadn't explored properly yet. It was like catching a whiff of something foul-smelling: No matter how much I wanted to will myself to breathe from my mouth and not inhale the aroma, at the last moment I always took deep, contemplative gulps. I had to *know*, even if the knowing was sickening.

So that was that. I'd try the massage place, and if I didn't like it, I'd quit and go back to Eros, or do more modeling. Then I'd know what it was like to touch men's bodies for money. I dialed the number and asked for an interview, dropping the name of my peep show coworker to make sure they'd know I wasn't a cop or a prankster.

The Temple of Shakti was located a few miles south of Seattle off the I-5 corridor, in a rundown little single-story house. The front yard was overgrown with clumps of brown grass. A hand-lettered sign on the door advised me to take off my shoes before entering. The letters were plump balloons, decorated by hearts and smiley faces. The sign had been written in Magic Marker, though the colors were faded from exposure. *A stripper made that sign,* I thought.

Boots in hand, my feet freezing in thin socks, I knocked on the door.

"Who is it?"

"Uh, it's me. I'm here for my interview." I spoke to the door, which remained closed.

"Oh! Great!" The locks jangled and the door flew open. A wall of heat pushed out at me. It was unbelievably solid, thick with moisture, saunaish. It felt good, though I couldn't believe customers didn't complain. It had to be ninety degrees in that house. I wondered if maybe I'd made a mistake, and the position they were hiring for actually involved Bikram yoga.

Inside, I put my boots down and stared at the woman who had opened the door.

"I'm Baby," she said, almost curtseying. "I'm so pleased to meet you!"

Baby was huge, a morbidly obese flesh mountain of a woman, as if someone had created an ordinarily fat lady and then decided not to stop. Rolls of fat bulged around her middle like stacked tires, defying gravity. She wore an immense pink sari that exposed the slack, loose hang of her belly. Her arms looked like enormous hams, sticking out helplessly from her body due to the monumental bulk of her torso. Her upper arms were approximately the size of my thighs.

In contrast to her massive arms, Baby's hands and wrists were ridiculously small: Her tiny, pudgy fingers looked like baby carrots.

Looking at Baby was like staring at an optical illusion—my mind kept refusing to accept how large she was, despite all evidence to the contrary.

She gazed at me, panting slightly with the effort of having opened the door. Her hair was wispy and reddish and stuck to her head in wet little curls. She had a bindi affixed to her forehead, slightly off-center. It gave her a disturbing, mongoloid look.

"Welcome to the Temple of Shakti!"

"Thank you," I said. "I'm so happy to be here."

"What's your name?" smiled Baby.

I hesitated. "Lily." I liked lilies. Plus flower names were kind of hippie-dippy. It seemed like that kind of thing would go over big here.

I wondered if Baby was ever going to let me in, or if she planned on conducting the interview on the porch.

"Come in, Lily," said Baby. "I'll show you the Temple!" She wrung her child-size hands in delight. It looked like she was choking something invisible.

We entered the main room from the foyer, passing several pairs of battered, forlorn-looking shoes. I put my boots against the wall, lining them up neatly, even though it looked like the other shoe owners had just kicked theirs off and let them fall randomly. A pair of Doc Martens sat next to a pair of men's dress shoes that looked scuffed and rundown at the heels. I was trying to get a sense of who else worked at the temple from the footwear in evidence, but Docs could belong to any kind of girl and the dress shoes obviously belonged to a customer.

Baby padded ahead of me, breathing audibly.

"Here in the Temple we believe in alignment of all the chakras," she said. "Do you know what a chakra is?"

I did, actually. "Those are the seven spots from the crown of the head down to the bottom of the spine that, uh, have something to do with, uh . . . ?"

"Yes!" crowed Baby. "Exactly! And we rub them all, and when they are properly manipulated the seeker feels a great sense of well-being, and often achieves release!"

Release. I got it. I'd spent about five years watching my customers "achieve release." The terminology was different, but it was a whole steaming load of the same old thing. I felt less off-balance, and more confident-slash-cocky. *I can do this.* A dick was a dick was a dick. I was in my milieu, despite the Eastern trappings.

The main room of the Temple held a couch and a few chairs. The couch faced an altar, which was arranged on a card table against one wall, under a poster of a grisly sexual position from the *Kama Sutra.* On the altar were statues of the Indian elephant god, and the Indian goddess with eight arms splayed out like a spider's legs, each hand holding something different or making a specific gesture. At the foot of each statue were dollar bills and coins. Central to the altar was a huge bowl of sand, with about a dozen sticks of incense pushed into the sand and standing up and out, like porcupine quills. They smoldered and dropped little ash turds onto the embroidered scarf that covered the card table. A dish of candy—butterscotch wheels and peppermint buttons— sat near the elephant god statue in a plastic Halloween-patterned bowl. I wasn't sure if the candy was part of the altar, or if it had just been set down there hastily by Baby when I knocked on the door. Most of the butterscotch wheels had been picked out, leaving far too many peppermint buttons behind. They looked dyed and inedible, their red and white swirl patterns appearing dangerous, like poisonous coloration.

Baby hustled past the altar. I noticed a kitchen, open to the main room of the Temple. Leaning against the counter was an older woman, with long gray hair tied in a horsey ponytail reaching almost to her waist. She wore stretch pants and an oversize Disney World T-shirt. Her face was plain and un-made up, with a strong hawkish nose and webs of wrinkles around her eyes and mouth. Her arms were folded and the corners of her mouth were turned down in focused concentration. She appeared to be microwaving something. Was she one of the workers? If so, working here was going to be a cinch.

I felt a slither of expectation in my stomach. All I'd have to do was wear makeup and a push-up bra, and customers used to the likes of the woman in the kitchen—and Baby—would line up to take sessions with me. Customers loved artifice, no matter how much they tried to pretend they were looking for sincerity; if they really wanted human connection and genuine goodwill, they'd be with their partners or trying to date nice, normal women, not purchasing adult entertainment from disaffected strippers. I'd found that I couldn't go wrong with a face full of peacock-colored makeup and an inch of satin fabric tucked between my ass cheeks, no matter the venue. My customarily whorish work appearance had been honed by years of pretending to be everyone's good-time girl. I didn't expect the Temple's client base to appreciate natural beauty more than any other group of horny, hooting primates would.

"That's Mommy," said Baby. "Hi, Mommy!"

"Hi, Baby," said the older woman. Her voice was low and resonant, like a cello. She sounded—tolerant? Resigned?

"Your mother?" I asked, surprised.

"Yes," said Baby. "She does our books. If you have any questions, though, just ask! Mommy will help you with anything you need to know. She knows everything!" Baby giggled. "And don't call her 'your mother.' Her name is *Mommy!*"

"Well, all right then," I said. "I'm very pleased to meet you, Mommy."

Mommy nodded. The microwave beeped. She opened the plastic door and took out a Cup O' Noodles. Shrimp flavor.

Baby grabbed my hand. "Lovely Miss Lily, I'm going to show you a practitioner's room. This is where we align the seekers' chakras, and open them to our healing energy! This way—" She led me into a brief hall with three closed doors and one open one. The open one was the bathroom. It looked clean enough.

Opening one of the doors, Baby said, "Go in, go in." I did, squeezing past a sheet-covered massage table.

The practitioner's room was meltingly humid, even more so than the main room of the Temple. A Crock-Pot sat in one corner, the orange light indicating it was on. It appeared to be full of water, which shimmered in the heat. The room was lit only by candles, which created a smoky haze and the heavy, churchy reek of burning wax.

"How does this all . . . happen?" I asked Baby. I meant, *How do we go from walking our clients past the altar and Mommy making lunch in the microwave, and get them up on the table, and start rubbing their dicks? Do we just bring them in and dive for their jocks?* I was really curious. I spied a boom box in the corner next to the Crock-Pot and wondered if I'd be expected to dance around before getting down to the cock-milking business. I hoped not. I was so sick of dancing sexily, making eye contact, and rubbing my body hungrily as if I actually wanted to get fucked. That was the whole point of being here at the Temple, and of turning fully illegal in general. I wanted to dispense with the charade that my work was motivated by my own blazing libido.

"Uh, how long does . . . this . . . usually take?" I couldn't think of a better way to put it. I was deeply ignorant about healing energy and chakra alignment. Not about the hand job part: I felt like I had that covered. But all the bells and whistles, all the faux-Indian stuff—that I didn't know anything about. I also didn't know if any of that mattered, here in the practitioner's room. Perhaps once the customer had been walked past the altar, all the fake Hindu stuff could stop and we could just do our jobs.

Baby said, "Why don't you take your clothes off and hop on the table?"

No. God, no. Please.

I looked at Baby. She was serious. She took a bottle of lotion from a side table and popped it into the hot water in the Crock-Pot.

In horror, I watched her begin to unwind her sari, folding it neatly as she unwrapped it from around her girth.

Oh, hell *no.*

And yet—

—that *thing* I had, that maddening itch of *needing to know*—it flexed like a fist, deep in my belly. And I realized that I was absolutely going to do this. I was going to get my chakras aligned by a behemoth named Baby while Mommy ate noodles in the kitchen outside the door.

I couldn't *not* do it.

I unbuckled my belt and let my boy-pants fall down. As I stepped out of them, I pulled my T-shirt over my head and tossed it to the floor.

I was wearing matching underwear—a black Wonderbra and a black satin thong—because I wasn't sure if I'd be asked to undress for scrutiny. My outer clothes were generally slobbish, but when going to a job interview I always made sure to be freshly shaven, body-sprayed, and clad in professional-caliber lingerie. Most adult industry managers expect strippers to arrive wearing loose, comfortable clothes and flat shoes, looking stocky and surly and possibly even lesbionic in boy-clothes. As long as you could whip them off and look like man-candy underneath, you'd be hired without any hesitation.

Baby was nude. I didn't look. I distracted myself by squatting down and folding my pants and T-shirt. I figured if I just squinted really hard whenever I looked Baby's way, all I'd see was a wall of indeterminate white flesh without alarming detail. I'd think of something that was bland and featureless, like mashed potatoes. Baby could be a big pile of mashed potatoes, and if I squinted, she'd stay mashed potatoes. About six hundred pounds worth, true, but still. It wasn't outside the realm of desperate possibility.

I pushed my folded clothes against the wall and clambered up onto the massage table gracelessly.

"Should I be facing up or down?" I screwed my eyes down tightly, turning my face toward Baby in an attempt to appear polite.

"Down, Lily!" Baby laughed. "It sounds like I'm talking to a dog, doesn't it? Down, Lily! Down, Lily!" She laughed again.

I lay on my belly, closing my eyes gratefully.

"Crazy Train"— Black Sabbath

When I felt Baby's tiny hands on my shoulder blades, I stiffened inadvertently. I wasn't much of a toucher, honestly. I didn't hug promiscuously. I didn't even like shaking hands much. I was less than fond of the idea of having my chakras rubbed by someone I'd just met—especially by someone who appeared to be completely insane—in a shabby little house masquerading as some kind of Indian palace. I forced myself to relax, though. I had to *know,* and obviously getting rubbed by Baby was part of the knowledge. It was unappealing, but no more so than a lot of the things I'd done for money. And, too, all I had to do was lie there and let it happen. I didn't even have to moan or thrash around.

I wondered if I'd get a butterscotch disc afterward, the way I used to get stickers after going to the dentist. Maybe Baby would make me take a peppermint instead, since there were so many more of those. I still wasn't sure if the candy was for mortals or not. Maybe it was some kind of Indian holy candy, tributes to the little statues like the incense and the coins. It looked like Brach's to me, but what did I know? Maybe the elephant god liked cheap drugstore candy. My guess was that Baby did, too.

The disorienting thing about Baby was that I couldn't tell what part of her body was touching me. As she ran her infant hands along my spine, Baby flesh pressed against my thigh. It was soft, yielding, and warm. Was it one of her belly rolls? Was it her breast? Was it a roly-poly arm? It was disconcerting not to know.

The cotton sheets under my face smelled good, like laundry detergent and Bounce. I guessed that even hippie temples used Bounce, which seemed incongruous, like the Cup O' Noodles Mommy was eating. Brand names seemed too modern, too American, too new to comfortably blend with the whole ancient temple ambience they had going on in the front room. But then again, this wasn't *really* a temple of any kind. It was a place men went to get their dicks jerked when they were too lazy or louche to do it themselves. The temple thing was just the frilly bow Baby and Mommy put on the whole package. Was it to make themselves feel better about what they were doing? Or was it some kind of legal dodge, maybe to gain tax immunity?

I heard a wet farty noise, and felt warm lotion on my back. Baby had retrieved the squeeze bottle of lotion from the Crock-Pot. It felt alarmingly seminal. I cringed.

"You're so knotted up," Baby said. "Are you stressed out, lovely Miss Lily?"

"No," I said. It sounded like a lie. I'd learned from experience that if you lied and it was totally obvious you were lying, you could tell the truth really quickly afterward and nobody would hold the first little lie against you. It was like the ten-second rule for dropping food—if you picked it up fast enough, the food didn't count as having hit the floor. "Yes. Sorry."

Baby giggled. "Well, we'll work out the kinks, Lily my love!"

"Great," I said. I was already sick of hearing my own name. I wished I had picked something else, something that didn't lend itself to alliteration so easily and obnoxiously.

As Baby worked, she explained the names of each chakra along my spine, and what each one supposedly represented. I wasn't paying much attention, but the top one, the head one, was allegedly the spiritual one, and the stomach one was ego, and the one opposite your crotch, kind of right above your butt crack, was sensuality and physical gratification. Baby said you had to rub all the chakras to "align" them, in order, starting at the head and going down to the bottom one. As she said this, she slipped a moist, lotiony finger between my ass cheeks and tapped. I almost screamed.

Despite that unexpected and unwelcome close call, though, it wasn't awful. With my clothes off, the room didn't feel overly warm. It was nice, womblike—a comfortable cocoon. If I hadn't been getting molested by Baby, I could imagine napping.

After about twenty minutes, Baby said, "Roll over, Lily! Roll over, girl! Arf arf!" It was safe to say I'd never been barked at by a six-hundred-pound heap of mashed potatoes before. Did she think she was being charmingly quirky? Was it possible that she suffered from Tourette's? It was hard to tell exactly *what* was wrong with Baby.

I complied, turning over and keeping my eyes squeezed shut. I was getting used to the idea of being nude in front of Baby, who was also nude, but I still didn't want to see her body, even if she could see mine.

It wasn't that I was prissy about bodies. I'd seen all kinds of male bodies, from the attractive to the shockingly ugly, from the young and fit to the appallingly broken. I'd seen rashes, herpes sores, warts, bumps, scars, scabs, hairy patches, fungal infections, lumps, piercings, bad tattoos, crusty shit-caked assholes, and pus-dripping cocks galore. My entire career was based upon tolerating an unceasing parade of bad health and poor hygiene.

I'd seen almost as many female bodies, those of my coworkers, in all stages of sanitation and undress. The realm of the physical didn't intimidate me. Once you've seen someone pull out a bloody, clotted tampon, piss herself, squeeze a zit, or fuck herself deep in the ass with a fist-sized toy, you kind of stop being freaked out about the weird and gross things bodies do. They're just bodies, and very few bodies are anything to write home about.

So it wasn't that I was frightened of seeing Baby naked. It was more that I hadn't been *paid* to see her naked, or to deal with her in such an intimate way, by having to look at her and pretend that her body was appetizing or at least not offputting. I had a game face, and I availed myself of it every day I worked shifts or modeled. But the idea of trotting that face out for free—because Baby had simply decided to be nude, because she *wanted* to be, instead of just saying, "Usually the practitioner does the session undressed," or whatever—that affronted me. She could be naked, if she wanted—it was *her* temple—but I didn't have to look.

I rearranged myself into a supine position on the massage table. My back felt warm and unpleasantly slimy from the lotion. I wondered how many cocks that lotion bottle had been used to lubricate. I squirmed around and tried to wipe some of it onto the sheet. *Intact skin is a barrier to HIV, hepatitis, viral STDs, and bacteria,* I told myself. I'd read that in a brochure I got from the Public Health Clinic downtown, a pamphlet encouraging gay men to masturbate onto each other or jerk each other off, instead of fucking or sucking. My back skin was intact. Therefore this was disgusting, but not technically dangerous. *Disgusting but not technically dangerous* seemed to be the motto for everything I'd done to earn money since I'd started working in the adult industry, actually.

Without warning, Baby slid her hands over my belly, up to my breasts.

"Whoa there!" I sputtered.

"Oh, sorry!" Baby laughed like a little girl, putting one hand over her mouth mischievously. Her fingertips left a smear of lotion on her upper lip. "Well, lovely Lily, at this point the practitioner rubs the front of the seeker. You have to get those chakras from the front, not just the back!" She looked disappointed. "You sure you don't want me to show you?"

"I think I pretty much have it," I said. "So, we rub the whole front of the . . . seeker. Ending up in the, uh, root chakra?" I was already getting the lingo. Not *cock,* not *prick,* not *dick*— *root chakra.*

"Yes, absolutely, Miss Lily! It is very spiritual for them. They often feel a great sense of relief when we get to the last chakra, once everything else has been perfectly aligned and adjusted."

I'll bet.

Baby trilled, "The whole adjustment takes about an hour. They can also book for an hour and a half, if they want an *intense adjustment."*

"Cool," I said. I opened my eyes, making sure to stare directly at the ceiling.

I had to admit, the whole temple setup was pretty brilliant. I mean, if I *had* been a cop, nothing illegal would have happened, or even been suggested. Baby had managed to train me to jerk men off for money according to house procedure, without ever once mentioning anything shadier than the root chakra.

My only question was, *Did Baby honestly believe she was running a temple, or did she know she was pimping girls out for holy hand jobs?*

"Can I get dressed now?"

"Yes you can, Miss Lily! Arf arf!" Blessedly, Baby shook the folds of her sari out and started winding the skirt part around her massive waist.

I rolled off the table and dressed quickly. Once I was in my pants and T-shirt, the room seemed hot again. It was hard to breathe because the still, close air was so heavily scented. Every breath was like inhaling a votive candle.

"How much does a one-hour, uh, adjustment cost?"

"One hundred and thirty. The temple keeps forty dollars, and the practitioner keeps ninety," Baby chirped. "Plus tips."

Tips? *She had to know.*

Once Baby was securely wrapped in her swaddling cloth, we exited the practitioner's room. Mommy was in the main room, reading a copy of *Star* on the couch. She looked up at us sharply as we came in.

"Miss Lily's all trained!" sang Baby.

"Are you?" asked Mommy, looking into my face. Her voice thrummed in my stomach chakra. Ego.

"Yes, ma'am—Mommy," I said. I sounded like a stutterer, or like I'd just called her Mammy, Al Jolson style. I imagined dropping to one knee and giving her a few rousing verses of "Swanee." Clearly, I had been unhinged by the cock-lotion backrub I'd just endured.

Mommy's eagle eyes didn't leave mine. "So, you understand about the chakra alignment, and the energy work we do here?"

"Yes ma'am," I said. "*Mommy.* Sorry."

She ignored my apology. "And you understand that you owe the house forty dollars for every hour session, and fifty for every hour and a half? And that there are no 'extras,' that we only provide *healing services* to seekers, not any kind of illegal activities?" Her lip curled when she said *illegal activities,* as if she were tasting something nasty.

The word *prostitution* hung between us like a cloud of nag champa. Neither of us said it.

This dame was balls-out. I kind of loved Mommy. She scared me, and I felt like attempting to bullshit her would be futile and ultimately humiliating. But I appreciated her hard-as-nails mien. Mommy was clearly the brains of the organization. If anyone knew what services we provided, and to whom, and how everything went down in those "practitioner rooms"—*really*—it was Mommy.

"Yes, ma'am, I understand," I said. It was as if Baby had dropped away and we were talking privately.

"Can you come in tomorrow, ready to work?" asked Mommy.

"What do I need?"

"Temple apparel—a sari, or a scarf, to tie around your hips. A simple top—tank top style, or long-sleeved. No T-shirts. Remember that this is *sacred space.*" I swore I saw a sneer brush over Mommy's stony features.

Was I actually going to do this?

Even as I wondered, I knew the answer was yes, I was. I had to know what it felt like to do what it was I had come to do. Leaving and not coming back would mean that I'd think about that stupid temple for the rest of my life, and feel like a coward.

"Personal items, makeup, essential oils that you like to use, whatever. Any CDs you'd like to play. We provide lotion, candles, incense, and clean laundry."

"Okay, got it," I said. "Thank you."

"Show up tomorrow at noon. You'll stay until six or so, if you work out," said Mommy.

"Who will I be working with?"

"Oh, you'll meet everyone tomorrow," said Mommy. Her eyes gleamed like wet rocks. Was she being cagey? Protecting the other girls—*practitioners*—until I'd proven that I wasn't a cop by doing a session myself?

"Cool," I said, quickly. I didn't want her to think I was trying to bust anyone, or get anyone's identity—even just their stripper names. *Practitioner* names. "I'll see you tomorrow, then, ma'a—Mommy."

Baby waved at me gaily. "Bye, Miss Lily!" she called, as I laced my boots in the foyer of the Temple and let myself out into the fresh, icy air.

"Love Is the Drug"— Roxy Music

I showed up at the Temple of Shakti the very next day with a big Indian cotton print scarf. I'd bought it at an import store downtown, before catching my bus out of Seattle to unincorporated King County. I'd also brought a packet of stick-on bindis just for fun, and to ingratiate myself with my new bosses. I hadn't wanted to wear a tank top, because my ink would've shown and I figured a bunch of tattoos wouldn't project the most sacred, templey image. Instead, I wore a plain black long-sleeved shirt that had enough spandex in it to hug my curves and show off all the eye-catching padding in my bra. I figured that by the time I was in the room with the customer, taking off my bra, he would already be naked and committed to the session. He might be a little let down that two of my cup sizes were actually made of cotton batting, but it wasn't like he was going to call the session off at that point. I'd seen that look of disappointment at the peeps, but nobody had ever walked off in a huff over my perfectly average bosom once he had his hard dick in his hand.

Or actually, in this case, in *my* hand.

In my backpack I had a big pump bottle full of hand sanitizer, a box of latex gloves, a bottle of water-based lubricant, makeup, a few CDs, and some raspberry body spray. I'd left my ID at home in case the Temple of Shakti got busted by Vice while I was in the building.

155

I let myself in through the rundown fence and picked my way over the sad brown clots of dead grass in the yard. As I bent over to remove my shoes on the porch, the front door flew open. I looked up, expecting Mommy or Baby. But it was a small, thin girl with a distinct overbite. She was pale, with long, straight black hair. She wore an Indian print skirt and a tiny little matching halter top. Her shoulders curved distinctly inward, making her tits hang in little cones.

"Hi," she said. "I'm Princess Lavender! I thought you were going to be my eleven-thirty!" Leaving the door open, she simply retreated into the Temple, as if it didn't matter to her whether I followed or not. Apparently I'd been right about the popularity of flower names at the Temple. But *Princess?* Her title seemed ostentatious and unnecessary. I briefly considered giving myself a royal honorific, too, but *Queen Lily* sounded like a great big boat and I didn't want to be outranked as a duchess or countess.

"I'm Lily," I said to her back. "I'm here to work."

"Oh yeah," said Lavender. "That's cool. Baby said she hired you yesterday."

"Uh-huh," I said.

"You have to do a session with me before you can do a solo session," Lavender said, frowning. She sighed deeply, then went over to the altar and scooped up a handful of coins, which she counted in her hand and then tucked into a pocket in her skirt.

"Bus fare," she said, when she saw me looking at her.

"Okay." I shrugged. "Is Mommy or Baby around?"

"They should be back in a little bit. We're just waiting for the dude who was supposed to show up here about ten minutes ago. I hate it when they're late." She sighed again, as if it were my fault the customer hadn't shown up on time. It wasn't like I had him bound and gagged on the porch. The guy was just *late.* I didn't see what the big deal was. Clients were often late to their own sessions. Some cheapskates even got off by booking time with a girl and then jerking off to the mere fact of having made an appointment with her, with no intention of actually showing up.

"I'm, uh, gonna go freshen up," I said. I grabbed my pack from the foyer where I'd left my shoes. The Docs and the dress shoes were still there. I wondered if they'd been abandoned, and if so, what size the Docs were. I needed new winter boots.

Lavender ignored me, so I walked past her to the bathroom. Maybe the chilly shoulder she was showing me was because the princess didn't care for commoners, or maybe she just wanted to be left alone with the spare change on the altar. I didn't care. I had no need to be Lavender's Best Friend Forever, as long as we could work together in détente. If she wasn't actively rude to me, I wouldn't tell on her for stealing quarters. There was also a chance that she was just having a crappy day and we'd gotten off on the wrong foot. Maybe we'd like each other better after doing a session together.

In the bathroom I put my wig on, caked a few layers of makeup on over my customary street amount, glued a rhinestone bindi between my eyebrows, and finished with a bright red coat of lipstick. It was weird to be barefoot instead of in high heels. I obviously couldn't wear my boots, and I couldn't just wear socks. I was glad I'd painted my toenails a few days ago.

Emerging from the bathroom, I heard voices—Lavender's lisp, and a lower voice—a man's. Was he our eleven-thirty? Both of them laughed, though I couldn't make out what they'd said that was so funny.

I threw my shoulders back, pushing my well-insulated tits out.

"Hi," I said, leaning against the door to the main room of the Temple.

Lavender whipped her head around, the smile quickly dropping from her face. The customer—*seeker*—stared past her narrow, birdlike shoulder, taking me in. I curled my lips up in what I hoped was a seductive—and yet still sacred—way.

"Hi," I said quietly. "I'm Lily."

"Lily is new," said Lavender, quickly.

The customer said, "Well, I'm pleased to meet you, Lily! How do you like it here so far?"

"I love it," I purred.

Lavender grabbed the customer's arm with an authoritative familiarity. "Let's go get settled in my room," she told him, force-marching him down the hall to a practitioner's room different than the one I'd been in the day before.

After a long time, Lavender emerged by herself.

"He's all settled," she said.

"Undressed?" I asked.

"Yeah. We can go in any time," she said. Her mousy little face looked perturbed.

"What's up?" I asked, meaning, *Is he going to be a problem?*

"Nothing," she said. "He's my regular. He's really nice."

Then I got it. Like most strippers, Princess Lavender was possessive of her regular clients. Nobody wanted a regular to see another girl, because the regular might like the other girl better. She was upset at having to do the session in conjunction with me, the new girl. It wasn't so bad when your regular saw another girl who wasn't cute, because that just made you look better by comparison. But if the girl he saw was attractive—particularly, if she was attractive in some way you weren't (I thought of Lavender's loose, pointy little breasts, versus my own round, super-padded ones)—then you risked losing your regular to the new girl. Men loved novelty. Even the most dedicated regular could jump ship at any time, swayed by the siren call of a brand-new inamorata. Most strippers guarded their regulars like cattle, herding them vigilantly and keeping them as far away from other workers as possible.

"How much do I get for this session?" I asked. "Do we split the ninety bucks?"

I tried to look as if I had no interest in stealing her regular. I didn't—not really. Besides, I couldn't do much about it, one way or the other. If Lavender's customer decided he was tired of her and wanted to start seeing me, there was nothing to do but take his money and hope that Lavender wouldn't hold his defection against me.

"No," said Lavender. "New girls only get twenty bucks for a duo." She paused. "You can ask Mommy if you don't believe me. It's for training."

Fuck. "That's cool," I said blandly. "But I'm not touching his cock for twenty."

"What?"

"I'm not touching his cock for twenty. I'll go topless and do some of the backrub, but I'm not touching dick for twenty bucks. That's ridiculous."

"Are you serious?" Lavender gazed at me incredulously.

"Listen, I know how to give a hand job, okay? I mean, a root chakra alignment thingie. I am not touching that man's cock for twenty bucks. You can tell Mommy if you want.

"And anyhow, he's *your* regular," I said. "If you finish him off, it's more likely he stays yours, right?"

I hoped that Lavender would find my logic inarguable. Twenty bucks barely bought you a tits-and-ass show at the peeps. I was incensed at the idea of actually breaking the law for so little money.

The idea of underpricing my labor was repellent in a deep and visceral way. It was contrary to everything I'd learned from the more experienced girls I'd worked with who'd given me the benefit of their knowledge freely, in the name of camaraderie and solidarity. To do this kind of work without feeling exploited, I'd learned, the provider absolutely needed to obtain as much money from the customer as she could, while performing the smallest amount of service. Reversing the equation was like handing your wallet to a mugger, and then voluntarily giving him your watch and your engagement ring, too. Nothing good ever came of being generous—it just made you feel foolish and used. Only suckers and amateurs had hearts of gold. Plus, giving clients more than they paid for taught them that they could bargain with us for lower prices, instead of giving us what we demanded without question. It was bad, bad precedent.

For ninety dollars, I was willing to milk a cock-teat to completion—I wasn't overly demure, and nearly a hundred bucks for an hour's easy work seemed fair. But for twenty, the customer was lucky to see my tits without a pane of cum-slathered glass between the two of us. I had standards. Not high ones—but they were intensely considered, and I was committed to them.

She shrugged. "Whatever," she said. "Come on."

We crept down the hall, and Lavender knocked softly at the closed door of her practitioner's room. Without waiting for a response, she opened the door and we both slipped inside.

It was so dark it was hard to see where the Crock-Pot was. The customer was a big, indistinct, towel-covered lump lying on his belly on the table. He didn't look up at us.

"Hi, Allan," cooed Lavender. "I'm here with Lily. Are you ready for us?"

Allan grunted.

I untied the scarf from around my hips and carefully removed my shirt, making sure not to pull my wig off with it. I decided to keep my bra and panties on for a while. Undressing was pointless if Allan was facing down, anyway. Besides, having lingerie on would give me something to do while Lavender jacked Allan off.

Princess Lavender had no such compunctions—she'd promptly stripped nude. I stared at her deflated, pancakey breasts and guessed she'd had a child or two. Her pubic hair was thick and ungroomed, creating a startlingly woolly triangle between her legs. She had a good ass, I thought. It wasn't too small for such a thin girl, and what she had was rounded and womanly. Her legs looked short and stubby, but only because I was used to seeing nude women in high heels—never flat-footed. Her toes were remarkably long.

Lavender seized the bottle of warm lotion from her Crock-Pot, and squeezed a generous amount onto Allan's hairy back. Then, instead of using her hands to rub it around, I was surprised to see her crawl up onto the table and lie full-length on top of him, writhing like a fish. Allan moaned.

So obviously, the whole "chakra alignment" thing was fairly flexible. Good to know.

As Lavender rubbed against Allan, she began whispering in his ear. Every now and again, she took his earlobe between her lips and bit it, or sucked on it. Eventually her tongue snaked out, and she began licking the side of his face like a cat. It was obscene, and fascinating. Doing what she was doing for under a hundred bucks was extraordinarily below scale. Customers paid nearly that much at Butterscotch's to masturbate in the presence of a lingerie-clad model, with absolutely no touching whatsoever. A hundred bucks at the peeps would buy you a brief toy show from a fully nude girl, but again, that was behind glass and there was no touching. Watching Lavender overperform for the money she was making from Allan was like watching a salesclerk ring up a diamond bracelet for the price of a candy necklace.

No wonder he's your regular, I thought. *He's getting the girlfriend experience for the price of a few lap dances.*

It occurred to me that Princess Lavender was not very smart.

After about fifteen minutes of foreplay, Lavender slid off her customer and faced me. Her front was greasy with cock lotion. It had matted her pubic hair. Wet ringlets stuck to her thighs.

"You do something," she hissed.

I approached Allan, reaching out like a sleepwalker. I probably looked like a little kid playing Frankenstein, but I couldn't see much and I didn't want to walk right into the table.

When my hands touched Allan's back, I started rubbing his shoulders vigorously, as if I were psyching him up to get back into the boxing ring. I realized I was rubbing too fast, that it probably didn't feel relaxing, and I forced myself to slow down.

"Is that you, Lily?" he asked.

"Sure is, sexy," I said. "Does that feel good?"

"Yeah," he said. "Why don't you get on top, like Lavender?"

Because I'm not a dumb whore with nothing else to offer but mileage, I thought. "Mm, Allan, I want to feel those strong, sexy traps of yours. Do you work out?"

It never failed.

"Yeah," he said. He stiffened a little in pride. "You can tell?"

"Oh, *yeah,*" I said. "Your back is rock hard." *If rocks were hairy, with moles and cystic acne.*

Lavender stared at me. I sensed she'd never thought of simply *talking* to a customer, running out his time with flattery, instead of crawling all over him and getting oil and customer skin cells all over herself. I'd learned to dirty-talk at Butterscotch's and honed my skills at the peeps. I was damned if I was going to touch Allan—or any "seeker"—any more than I absolutely had to. If I did it right, they'd never notice the difference.

"You know what would really turn me on, Allan?" I asked, running my fingertips up and down his back idly.

I didn't wait for him to respond. "What would really, *really* turn me on would be to watch sexy little Lavender *adjust your chakras,* nice and hard and nasty, baby."

". . . Really?" Allan was breathing harder.

"Yes," I whispered. "Lavender is such a hot, naughty girl. She was just telling me how much she loves adjusting your chakras in the other room, before we came in."

I checked the timer on the boom box. We'd been in there for a little over half an hour. He'd paid for an hour. I assumed Lavender gave her customers their full time, unlike most other working girls who'd short any client who wasn't a clock-watcher. I didn't think she did it because she was honest—I figured the idea of shorting her clients probably just hadn't occurred to her. Rushing the clock was like talking to them, using words instead of touch or physical performance—less work for the same price. Only tragically stupid working girls knocked themselves out for their customers if they didn't have to.

". . . Really? You want to watch, Lily?"

"Oh, *yeah*," I said. I leaned down and blew lightly in one hairy, wax-plugged ear. *Ugh*. I couldn't believe Lavender had licked that. What was *wrong* with her?

"Time to turn over!" said Lavender, clapping her hands. Both Allan and I jumped.

"She Goes Down"— Mötley Crüe

Lavender whisked Allan's towel off, exposing his wide, flat buttocks. Groaning, he used his arms to push himself up and onto one meaty hip. Then he rearranged himself, faceup, on the massage table. His face looked puffy from having been upside down for so long. He blinked up at us greedily, looking from me to Lavender as if trying to commit our bodies to memory, or maybe just trying to figure out which one of us was going to make the first move toward his cock. He was semihard already, with a string of cock drool connecting the tip of his dick to his own hairy belly.

I checked the timer on the boom box again: We had about twenty minutes to bring this home. Easy. I could waste twenty minutes of any customer's time in my sleep, then all Lavender would have to do was give his dick two or three firm pumps and Allan's chakras would be properly aligned, giving him the "deep sense of relief" he was paying for.

Princess Lavender climbed up on the table again, kneeling on all fours with her woolly pussy directly over Allan's face and *her* face a few inches from his lurching crotch, in a classic sixty-nine. I wondered again what the hell she was doing. Was it possible she was showing off for me, the new girl? Trying to impress me with how "good" her sessions were? Or was she making absolutely sure that Allan, her regular, wouldn't forsake her, if in fact she was his primary provider?

Seizing Allan's dick in both hands, Lavender pressed her overbite to his shaft, blowing against his skin and planting soft, goldfishy kisses on his balls. Suddenly my stomach cramped into a tight cold fist, and I couldn't breathe. *Bare oral? For ninety bucks?* I felt like covering my own eyes. She wasn't sucking his cock per se, but the kissing was almost worse. That broke two working-girl rules at once: No kissing, and no giving the customer more than he's paid for. Lavender's transgressions were obscene. My face burned in secondhand shame, as if my bindi were melting off or maybe bursting into flames. I needed air; I needed to get the hot, heavy wig off my head. I felt implicated just by watching.

What did any of this have to do with "energy work"? This was just straight-up whoring, with no fake ayurvedic stuff to soft-pedal the sexual nature of the transaction. The Princess could do whatever she wanted, but if I was going to be expected to kiss dick, I was walking. There was no way I was doing that, no matter how the other girls made their money at the Temple.

Lavender continued kissing and blowing on Allan's balls while stroking his cock with her hands. She had become a living pocket pussy, a super-deluxe girl-shaped jack-off device made of flesh and bone—the porn version of a Fisher-Price busy box. Like the eight-armed goddess on the altar, her hands and mouth and crotch and ass were somehow everywhere on Allan, rubbing and patting and pulling and blowing and kissing and licking. She was multitasking. It was the most demented thing I'd ever seen any working girl do for pay, and I thought I'd seen every perversion of decency possible. She was an octopus made of holes and fingers: a fucktopus.

The thing was—you can crawl in the gutter, stand up, brush yourself off, and laugh at what you've just done to pay your rent if you know the gutter isn't where you really belong. You can fuck yourself with toys and fake-masturbate and model and pretend to be an insatiable fantasy girl if you know who you really are, in all your smartness and silliness. That you're still the you who grew up and went to school and read books and ate food and cried and had crushes and friends and pets and a whole history of being a real, live person. If you can change right back into yourself and leave the fantasy girl image behind the second you're done working, then you can protect the kernel of your actual personhood from all the people who prefer to consider you a living cum repository.

But Lavender was not only in the gutter, she was rolling in rot and gobbling it up as fast as she could, becoming a debased thing with no boundaries between herself and the filth that surrounded her. It was as if Lavender had shed her humanity—and every bit of her self-respect—along with her skirt and halter top. I couldn't imagine her laughing about this session afterward, or even seeing anything about it that was funny at all. She was selling herself out. It made me feel like crying, or throwing up.

Oh well, it was her decision. I had to stop thinking about it or there was no way I could finish our session. I thought of Scarlett O'Hara, saying *Fiddle-dee-dee, I'll think about it tomorrow!* Except I wasn't going to think about it tomorrow, or ever again, hopefully. If I thought about it, I was pretty sure I'd never be able to look at a customer again without wanting to saw his dick off with a serrated steak knife. I couldn't afford to think about it.

I couldn't help but notice Allan sniffing Lavender's pussy, which made sense because it was only about half an inch away from the tip of his nose. I wondered if it was malodorous, due to her massive pubic bush. I knew it was just hair, but a hairy crotch just didn't seem *clean* to me anymore after five years of meticulously shaving my own. I had to hand it to Lavender for leaving herself natural, though. It was rare to see a stripper without rashy, red razor bumps in the creases of her inner thighs. The bumps were ugly and we all had them. I covered mine with makeup sometimes, and other times I just let them hang out as punishment to the men jerking off to me. They didn't care either way. Most of them would be masturbating to their own dogs' assholes if they weren't paying to look at mine—I was merely a slightly nicer, slightly more luxe series of warm wet holes.

I shuddered as I observed Allan growing bolder, nuzzling Lavender's crotch hair with his lips and nose. His cock was fully erect now—flushed and angry, like a pimple. I figured that if Lavender squeezed it, it would burst and splatter cum all over his belly and her face. Watching her manipulate Allan's dick was like watching someone play Russian roulette. I was horrified, but I couldn't look away.

I had to do something. I had to stop caring about Lavender and her inexplicable desire to overserve her customer. That had nothing to do with me; it was her business. But I couldn't just stand there barefoot in that sweltering little room, doing nothing. I had to expedite this scene. I was a professional.

"Does that feel good, Allan?" I whispered.

He moaned, and farted. It sounded like a long, drawn-out trumpet note, midrange, with a wistful and evocative fade.

Lavender jerked her head back from his crotch. "Thanks a lot!" she snarled at me.

Oh yeah, because I made him fart, Princess. If you weren't slurping up his nuts like spaghetti, you wouldn't have gotten a faceful of gas, idiot.

"Sorry," said Allan, sheepishly. "I had Chinese for lunch."

"Oh no, Allan, don't worry, baby!" I said. "A good chakra alignment is like a massage—it moves everything around inside you, and sometimes churns up a little air." I had no idea if this was true or not. I was sorry that he'd broken wind in Lavender's ratlike little face, but I hoped it would inspire her to dismount.

No such luck. Lavender merely shifted, and sat on Allan's chest reverse cowgirl style, plucking at the stem of his cock. She stared at me and made a circling gesture with one finger, as if she were describing the movement of hands on a tiny clock. *Get on with it, whatever it is you're doing,* the gesture said.

Because I couldn't think of anything sexy to say to follow up my discussion of energy-work-induced flatulence, I stalled by sighing like a porn star. "*Ooooooooooooooooooh,* yeah, Allan. Looking at that hard cock of yours is getting my pretty little pussy all wet."

"It is?" Allan gasped. "Can I feel your hands on me? Can you kind of take turns?"

"*Ooooooooooooooooooh,*" I said again, stalling while I tried to think of how to gracefully avoid touching Allan's leaking prick.

Lavender said, "Yeah, Lily. Why don't you take a turn? I know how turned on you get when you start *aligning the root chakra.*"

Bitch! So that was how she was trying to get her revenge for the fart. Which hadn't even been my fault. I'd felt sorry for her! I'd mourned her humanity! I was incensed. Anger ate up the sadness in my chest. It felt cool and minty and refreshing.

"Maybe I just will, Princess Lavender," I said. "Mmmmmmmmmmm! But let me get out of this naughty, sexy lingerie first. Would you like that, Allan?"

He nodded rapidly. His cheeks were red in two distinct spots. He looked like a tin soldier.

I turned around modestly. Men loved that—it made any stripper seem more like a real girl, and less like a paid professional. Then I slowly unhooked my Wonderbra and slid the straps down over my arms, counting *one one thousand, two one thousand, three one thousand, four one thousand, five one thousand* as I did so. I sneaked a peek at the timer. Ten more minutes.

Leaving my thong on, I turned toward Allan and Lavender. I'd always been proud of my tits. They weren't overly large, but they were grapefruit-size—natural Ds—and more importantly, they still defied gravity. In contrast to Lavender's desiccated, sucked-out flesh-sacks, my breasts were round and firm and pretty. I put my hands under them, lifting them slightly.

Allan's cock pulsed.

"Oh, I want to lick those titties, Lily," he said. He farted again—another mellow, sustained coronet note. It was like he was a jazz farter, taking center stage for his solo. "Sorry! It's the Chinese. I knew I shouldn't have had it."

He pushed his hips upward, thrusting his cock into Lavender's hands, enthusiastically fucking her cockjuice-slicked palms.

"Are you ready for your seventh chakra release, sugar?" I asked, still holding my own breasts. I was convinced that holding them up as much as possible kept them firm. Also, with my hands full, nobody could expect me to serve Allan his creamy vanilla shake. That was all on Lavender—Miss Ninety Bucks could take the hit. It was clear she wasn't fazed by heavy customer contact anyway. I reminded myself to feel mad, not sad. I wasn't like Lavender, and I didn't want to be. I had to stay separate. I had to remember that I was *real,* not a living fuck-doll.

I thought again about Lavender's mouth on Allan's drooling cock. *Herpes!* my mind sang gaily. *Oral, and genital! Transmitting! Maybe even switching places, do-si-do!* I wasn't sure which was grosser, the fact that Lavender didn't care about getting a disease from Allan, or the fact that Allan didn't care about getting a disease from Lavender. Maybe they were just two filthy people who viewed incurable sexually transmitted diseases as casually as most people viewed paper cuts or the common cold. I had never had an STD, but maybe once you got one, you stopped being so vigilant. Or maybe the whole "spiritual" packaging of the Temple made something as worldly as condoms seem superfluous.

I made deliberate, sultry eye contact with Allan, while tweaking my own nipples. "Oh," I said. "Yes. I want you to come for me, baby."

Lavender shook her head furiously. *Release,* she mouthed at me.

"I mean, I want you to achieve release for me, honey. Can you do that for me?" *Get ready, Princess. You're gonna get a handful of man-batter in about five seconds.* I was sick of this session—sick of working with Lavender, sick of Allan breaking chicken chow mein–scented wind, sick of standing there topless.

The whole thing—the Temple setup, the session, Lavender's artless nudity, my alarming wig, *everything*—was shoddy. It was even a second-rate sin—a hand job, not even a fuck. I wanted to go home.

"*You want me to do it now?*" Allan croaked. His balls had drawn up tight against his body. The wet rasp of his wheezing filled the room.

Lavender leaned back, holding his prick at arm's length. I took a big step backward, picking up and holding my bra in my hands protectively. I thought of cop-show terminology: *We have a shooter!*

I hoped with all my heart that Allan was more of a dribbler. I couldn't handle seeing much cock-snot at this point. I already suspected I was losing my mind—I was certain that a big porn-style money shot on Allan's part would result in me throttling him to death. If any of his waste got onto my skin or costume, I planned on stabbing his eyes out with one of the plastic forks Mommy kept on the kitchen counter for her noodles. I could almost hear his screams, could almost feel the fork lodged securely in my hand as I brought it down, again and again.

It occurred to me that I probably needed counseling.

"*Unnnngh! Unnngh!*" Allan bucked on the table, depositing droplets of semen into Lavender's hands. I waited until he was done, then I put my Wonderbra back on, hooking it carefully behind my back. Then I replaced my Spandex shirt and retied the scarf around my hips.

Once I was completely clad, and after checking my wig to make sure it was still pinned on straight, I took a Bounce-scented washcloth from a little folded pile of them next to the Crock-Pot and presented it to Lavender. She snatched it from me and used it to wipe Allan's cum from her hands and arms, before hopping off the massage table and retrieving a few more washcloths for herself. I noticed she dipped them into the hot, lotiony Crock-Pot water before she used them to clean herself.

Allan lay there, his cum slowly turning transparent and drying on his belly.

"Well!" I said brightly. We all breathed. We'd all lived through what had just happened. My hands were claws at my sides. I forced myself to relax. We were done.

Lavender turned to Allan and said, "We'll give you a few moments to get dressed." Her Indian print skirt and matching halter top were bunched up in her hands. Without looking at me, she marched over to the door, her small, high buttocks grinding together like pebbles. At the open door, she turned back. "Leave your donation on the table, Allan, just like always, okay?"

He grunted in assent, and heaved himself up to a sitting position. He wouldn't meet my eyes, but that wasn't unusual. Usually after coming—*achieving release*—customers couldn't leave fast enough. They certainly didn't want their dairymaids to attempt small talk. Pursuing conversation after a session—even innocently, in the interest of appearing gracious—had earned many an inexperienced stripper sudden frightening flashes of rage from clients who were ashamed of their appetites, or of having paid for sexual service, or of having been unfaithful to their loving, oblivious partners. It was best to let them dress and exit the premises as rapidly as they wanted to.

I left the room silently, shutting the door behind myself.

So that was that. I'd done it. I hadn't touched him, but I'd been in the room for Lavender's prostitution; if he'd been a cop, I would have gotten a free ride to King County lockup, too—an identical ticket and the same charges. Vice didn't differentiate between whores who touched dick for money and whores who just agreed to touch dick for money. Me being in the room would be considered a distinct and enthusiastic agreement to any cop worth his nickel-plated badge.

How did I feel?

I didn't know. I was pretty sure I didn't feel bad, though, now that it was over.

Was the Temple tolerable? I thought so. I didn't know everything, and I hadn't done my own session yet, but I had the general idea. Yes, it was bad. But, as disgusting as the work was, I felt a flutter of interest, of professional challenge. There had to be an angle, a way to make money here by using my skills and avoiding Lavender's tragic overservice.

I was still real.

Twenty bucks for a few minutes of topless dirty talk had turned out to be acceptable. When I did my own sessions—if I decided to come back—I'd be earning ninety. There wasn't a single terrible Christmas decoration to be seen anywhere in the Temple. And the odor of incense and burning wax beat the smell of Taya's piss, hands down. I was already pretty accustomed to the smell of semen.

Lavender was dressing hastily in the hallway.

"You did a really good job," I said. "I can see why he's your regular."

She looked at me uncertainly, surely wondering if I was mocking her.

"Dude, I'm serious. Thanks for letting me sit in."

"Whatever," said the Princess, tossing her lank black hair over her shoulders.

I shrugged.

Then she said, "He'd better tip."

After a moment, Lavender added, "I'll split the tip with you, if there is one."

I smiled at her, surprised by her kindness. I didn't want to hate Lavender. I didn't want her to hate me. I wanted us to be real together, for Lavender to morph from a busy box of cunt and ass and mouth to . . . I wasn't sure. I tried on *a friend.* It didn't feel quite right. *A comrade?* That was closer.

In spite of everything—my anger, my disgust, my fleeting homicidal rage—we working ladies needed to stick together. If we wasted our time being mean to each other, the customers could divide and conquer and get whatever they wanted from us. It was a slippery slope from that to ball-kissing. Clients had to be aware they were dealing with a united front, or they'd use us like Kleenex. Ultimately, weren't we all whores in the eyes of the law and also to most of the rest of society?

I reminded myself to try really, really hard to be nice to Lavender in the future. Maybe we'd never be friends, but we needed to have each other's backs.

"Awesome. Thank you," I said.

"We should walk him out," said Lavender, tying her halter behind her skinny neck. She bit her nail.

I couldn't help noticing that she hadn't bothered to wash her hands after her session. I winced.

On our way back to Lavender's practitioner room to let Allan out, I asked her about her choice of words—"donation," she'd said, not payment.

"Yeah, always say *donation,*" said Lavender. "If Mommy hears you say *payment* you get in trouble." We both fell silent, thinking about being in trouble with Mommy. Mommy's wrath seemed like it would be terrifying, somehow, even though I'd only seen her eat noodles and read celebrity magazines. It was her watchfulness—it inspired a dreadful sense of free fall.

"Okay, so they *donate* after the show?" I asked, incredulously. "Not before?"

"Nuh-uh," said the princess. "If they donate before, that's prostitution because they're paying for services. They have to put down the money after because they're *donating* to the Temple, get it?"

Fuck me. Trust a customer to pay me *after* he'd had his orgasm? It was outlandish, and unprecedented. You always got your money up front—always. It was like kissing—but I guess if some customers could get their nutsacks kissed here, other rules could be broken, too.

I had to be polite, though. "That, uh . . . works? They really do pay afterward?"

Lavender stared at me. "*Very occasionally* we get stiffed. But most seekers want to come back."

I could see that. Who wouldn't want Cadillac service for the price of an old primer-studded Pinto? *Well, kiss my balls! I'm getting jerked off on a sliding scale!*

I didn't know whether to guffaw, or sob.

"Lucky and Unhappy"— Air

We walked Allan out to the foyer, where Lavender kissed him on the cheek and gave him a long, tight hug. When he turned to me with his arms outstretched, I quickly stepped back and punched him lightly on the shoulder. "Come see us again, champ," I said, pitching my voice low and sexy.

Once Allan was safely out the door, Lavender flopped onto the couch opposite the altar. After a moment of uncertainty—*Would I be welcome?*—I followed her and sat primly at the other end of the couch.

"So that's pretty much how it goes?" I asked. "Aren't you gonna check to make sure he left his *donation?*"

"He left it," said Lavender. "He's been seeing me for years." She fanned herself with one hand, like a mediocre actress portraying one of Tennessee Williams's elegant, faded-magnolia heroines. The gesture looked contrived, like something Lavender had seen on TV.

I couldn't stand it. "Uh—I have a question."

"Yeah?"

"Okay," I said. I had to think really hard about how to phrase this without insulting Lavender and without sounding like a dirty, money-minded stripper instead of an ethereal, chakra-aligning healer. I wasn't sure how much the princess bought into the whole

Temple charade, so I had to err on the side of caution—what if she reported back to Mommy directly after our session? Anything I said could get me fired, I assumed, and I'd already made a stand about not touching cock for twenty bucks. I was not only skating on thin ice, I was stomping on it. But still, I had to ask.

"Okay. So, uh, I noticed you, uh . . . put your mouth on Allan's *root chakra*. Well, not the chakra exactly, not the head of the chakra, but on the uh, his . . ." *Testicles. Nutsack. Balls.* "On his—near the *base* of his root chakra."

"Yeah?" Lavender stared at me. Even with her mouth shut, I could see her front teeth. She didn't seem to have enough upper lip to keep them covered.

A mean little voice in me whispered, *Maybe Lavender does this kind of work because she's too ugly to strip.* I was mildly shocked at my own cruelty. It wasn't like she hadn't offered to split Allan's tip with me, even after I'd refused to touch his weenie. And just because she'd let him sniff her pussy, that didn't make her a bad person. After all, with all that hair, she was practically wearing wool bikini panties anyway.

But no—*nobody* was too ugly to strip. I'd worked with all kinds of women, from the magazine-gorgeous to the frankly unattractive. Lavender could make money as a stripper if I could. Her rabbity front teeth were no worse than my chunky legs. Neither of us looked like fashion models—I had tattoos on my arms and cellulite on the backs of my thighs; Lavender was more Bugs Bunny than Playboy Bunny. She had to be here because she wanted to be.

I guessed we both were.

"Okay. So you put your mouth there, that's totally fine—I'm not trying to judge. I'm just curious about, um, STDs? Herpes? Stuff like that? Aren't you scared of getting something from a seeker, doing the kind of . . . stuff we do?"

Lavender rolled her eyes at me. "I've done my research," she said. "The human mouth kills all viruses and bacteria. Nothing can live in that kind of body heat. Everything dies," she concluded.

"Plus, the only way you get sick is if you're conflicted about being a healer, like if you feel guilty or dirty. And I don't. So I've got nothing to worry about."

Apparently Princess Lavender had her mouth confused with a hospital-grade autoclave. I wondered where she'd done her research, or if by *research* she meant she'd paged through a few issues of *Penthouse Forum* from the early '70s, before anyone had heard of anything more injurious than the clap—when all you had to do was take antibiotics for a week after a regrettable sexual encounter and you were as good as new.

Dear Penthouse,
I never thought this would happen to me, but I'm completely immune to all forms of sexually transmitted disease! So I lick customer nutsack and don't bother washing my hands after sessions!
Signed, A Healer

It was like hearing that her birth control method was douching with Pepsi, post–intercourse. Or that she honestly believed the earth was flat. It was a display of such astonishing ignorance that I didn't even know where to start, or what words we could possibly define similarly. It was like realizing that someone you'd been talking to for hours, who had been animatedly shaking her head in agreement and laughing at all your jokes, actually didn't speak a work of English.

"Uh, yeah," I said. "But actually, herpes is a skin-shed virus that's usually without symptoms. That means just rubbing your mouth on someone's junk—even if there's no lesion, just from the skin cells—you can get, you know . . . *herpes.*"

Lavender frowned at me. "Well, I'm not worried. I'm not going to get anything from the customers," she said. "Maybe *you* have to worry about that stuff. But I'm a healer, not a prostitute." She stared at me. She didn't have to call me a whore.

The fact that I was worried about universal healthcare precautions marked me as one, and we both knew it.

"So you're seriously . . . okay with everything?" I couldn't stand it. I was waiting for her to point her finger at me, laugh, and say, *Wow, I really got you! You really thought I was that stupid!* Then maybe we could both laugh and I could deep-breathe until my heart stopped crashing against my own rib cage like it was trying to escape.

"*Yes,*" she said, annoyed. "I'm clean. Besides, it's not like we're having *sex* with them."

No, we're just getting their nasty bodily fluids and skin cells and shed viruses all over ourselves. I shuddered. Maybe I could sneak into the bathroom after every session to scrub myself and spray myself down with bleach water. Was there any way I could convince my clients to wear condoms for their root chakra alignments? My mind raced.

Lavender hopped up and went over to the fridge. She took out a liter of Evian, twisting the top off and taking a big, thirsty swig of the cold water. "Want some?" she asked, holding the bottle out toward me, licking a stray droplet of water from her lower lip.

I managed not to shriek. "Uh, no thanks, but thank you," I said. She could keep her herpes water to herself. I made a mental note to bring my own bottle of water, and to hide it somewhere Princess Lavender of the Autoclave Mouth could never, ever find it.

All of a sudden I thought of Eros Galaxy, and the sweet, sweet glass between the customers and myself. Sure, it was uncomfortable and humiliating being penned up in a plastic kennel, waiting for customers to drop dollar bills into my booth in order to purchase clinical views of my pussy in minute-long increments. But at least all their disease and filth stayed on their side of the glass. Here, I would be making more—and performing less, I hoped—but the flip side was, I'd be touching their semen. There was no way around it. I'd be touching it. *Disgusting, but not technically dangerous,* I tried to tell myself. The reality was, though, that if I got a speck of dust in my eye, I wouldn't be able to rub it until I got home and disinfected myself first. It gave me pause.

"I'm gonna go clean my room," said Lavender.

"Cool, I'll come with," I said. I didn't want her pocketing the tip she'd promised to split with me. Plus, I wanted to see how to get the practitioner room back into shape for the next customer. Seeker.

We entered the room to the unmistakable, sulphury scent of egg rolls. Lavender threw the door open and flicked on the lights. "Pee-ew," she said. She swung the door open and shut rapidly, using it as a giant fan to disperse the stench. I spied a pile of bills on the table. He'd paid! I realized I hadn't really believed he would. I felt a small rush of relief.

This would be dicey. "Should I count it, Lavender?" I asked. I was getting awfully close to one of the things you never, ever do, which was touching another girl's money. But twenty of it was mine, so I felt bold enough to ask.

"Yeah, sure," she said. She stripped the greasy, lotion-stained sheet off the massage table and straightened the bath towel that lay underneath—to pad the table and soak up any excess cock oil, I supposed. I noted that she didn't bother to change the towel; she just draped a fresh cotton sheet over it. Apparently the seekers couldn't get anything from *each other* in the Temple, either—not crabs, not ringworm, and not any other communicable disease spread by lying sprawled out nude on the same essentially unchanged linens. That, like the Temple practitioners' immunity to herpes and hepatitis, was also good to know. All the years I'd spent worrying about things like hygiene—only to be schooled by Princess Lavender, who had done her research and found that all the diseases other people got couldn't be transmitted in a rundown hippie house doubling as an Indian temple.

I snatched up Allan's money and counted it onto the massage table as Lavender bustled around, blowing out candles and turning off the boom box and Crock-Pot. He'd paid his $130 for his hour session, plus the extra $20 for me—*Good boy*—and left us an extra $20. Not bad. Not good, but not insulting. "Hey, we each got ten," I said.

"Cool," she said.

Outside the practitioner room, I heard a key rattling in the front door, and suddenly, the foyer exploded with activity and noise. It was Baby and Mommy, both carrying brown paper sacks of groceries, both chattering loudly and talking over each other. Baby was gasping with laughter, or with the exertion of moving her bulk from the front entrance into the Temple proper. I froze at the sink, unsure of what to expect. Were the practitioners even allowed in the kitchen? Or was that Mommy's territory? Would my long-sleeved spandex T-shirt pass muster? Was my wig too hookery? Was Lavender going to tell on me for not touching Allan's dick?

"Lovely Miss Lily!" laughed Baby. "Arf arf! You look beautiful! Is that a wig? I could barely tell! Did you do your session with Lavender? How did it feel to heal a seeker? Lavender, how did she do?" Her words rumbled out, stacking on top of each other, fighting each other for emphasis, as if everything she said were italicized. Between phrases, Baby fought for breath.

Lavender stared at me. "She did great," she said slowly.

Thank you, Princess—I owe you one. "I learned a lot," I said. "It was—good. It was fine." *I learned that only dirty, guilty people contract STDs. And that Lavender has a mouth hot enough to can fruit. And that the ayurvedic phrase for* balls *is* the base of the root chakra. Come to think of it, I really had learned a lot.

Mommy gazed at Lavender. "Did you drop your forty dollars to the house, Lavvie?" she asked, her voice suddenly businesslike.

"No. Here," she said, handing Mommy two twenties. "Lily, here's yours." She pressed twenty dollars into my hand. "I'll give you your ten as soon as I get some change."

I nodded.

Mommy looked at me. "You have a four o'clock solo session. Do you feel confident about working by yourself?"

I did, actually. I figured I'd have a better chance of running the session my way without Princess Lavender there orally autoclaving my client's dick. I imagined myself running out my client's time with a mediocre backrub and a lot of flattery, and then giving him the secret Masonic handshake in the last few moments of the session. Then I'd wash my hands for ten more minutes, and maybe even see if I could find any household cleansing products I could dilute and use as a final germ-killing rinse. It was all good. It beat pulling my labia apart with my fingers and watching customers frantically jerk themselves off like spider monkeys, spraying hot ropes of cum all over the glass that separated their cocks from my body.

"Yes, Mommy," I smiled.

Lavender tossed me a sharp look. Her little ferret face was unreadable.

For the next three hours, Baby did our horoscopes, using a complicated chart from a big book with pictures of constellations on the front cover. I wasn't sure how astrology fit into traditional Hinduism, but it was clear that Baby felt no conflict in her interests. The phone rang every now and again. Mommy answered it from the kitchen in her deep, warm voice, where she was making a pot of Kraft macaroni and cheese and leafing through this week's *People* magazine. I felt her eyes on me every now and again, and when I did, I made sure to keep my head down.

"She's Crafty"— Beastie Boys

At ten till four there was a hesitant knock at the front door of the Temple. My head jerked up. It figured that my client would be early, appearing before I'd freshened my makeup or retied my scarf. I hoped he didn't think I'd be giving him ten extra minutes of *healing touch*. He was going to be lucky if I gave him forty minutes total. Lavender may have been a healer, but I was a stripper, a model, and an adult entertainer. It was against my religion not to short a client as much as humanly possible.

Mommy made an emphatic brushing motion with both her hands, as if to say, *Answer the door! Go get him!*

Baby and Lavender melted away into a practitioner room and the bathroom, respectively. I noticed that Baby shoved the astrology book under the altar as she exited the main room. I wondered what else was under there, hastily cached whenever someone knocked on the door. More Halloween candy? A copy of the *I Ching*? Ten crucifixes? A bloody, severed goat's head? Anything seemed possible.

I crept to the door on my bare feet, feeling short and top-heavy in my wig, padded bra, and complicated makeup. I felt like a television newscaster, wearing a suit and tie on top and shorts underneath the broadcast desk, where they wouldn't show. I still wasn't used to walking flat-footed. It was a little better when I walked on tiptoe as if I were wearing invisible heels, like a ballerina mincing across the stage *en pointe*.

I opened the door to reveal my four o'clock. He was average in nearly every way. To tell you the truth, after so many years, I was less likely to recognize a client by his face than I was to recall him by his penis and his sexual proclivities. I was pretty sure I hadn't seen this man at Butterscotch's or Eros, but I wouldn't know for sure until he'd stripped and gotten hard. He stood awkwardly on the threshold, perched as if considering a hasty retreat back to the safety of his car.

"Hello, darling," I said, smiling and seizing his hands. *Ha, try to escape now!* I held them tightly, making deliberate eye contact. *Your ass is mine, bitch.* "I'm Lily. I'm brand-new," I said shyly. "Have you been here before?"

"No," my customer said. That didn't mean much. They loved to lie about their adult entertainment recidivism.

"No!" I said, delighted. "Well, I guess we're both . . . shiny and new, then, right?"

"Yeah," he said. He made no move to come into the foyer, so I gave his hands a good yank. He stumbled forward, then regained his balance.

"Hey," he protested.

"Oops, sorry," I giggled, slipping behind him and locking the door. "Why don't you take your shoes off, darling? Welcome to the Temple of Shakti!"

Cornered, he stooped to slip off his loafers. Before he could straighten up, I seized his upper arm and force-marched him into the main room of the Temple.

I'd had countless customers make appointments with me at Butterscotch's, either for lingerie shows or for domination sessions, and one of the things a large number of them liked doing was showing up for their appointments—thus getting a good look at me, dressed for our session in my lingerie or fetish wear—then making hasty excuses and leaving, to blatantly jerk off for free in their cars outside. It was incredibly annoying and could also be financially disastrous, if you'd booked your client for two hours and turned down other potential customers for that time slot. So there was no way I was letting this client out of my grasp for more than a few seconds. Temple or not, I was there to make money. So far I'd only made twenty bucks—thirty, if you counted the ten-dollar tip I was supposed to get from Lavender by the end of the day. Those wages were laughable for doing something that could get me arrested. Sin was supposed to pay, and pay well—not just grudgingly make ends meet if you clipped coupons and never went shopping.

"What's your name, gorgeous?" I asked my customer, who seemed dazed by the intense heat of the Temple, and slightly sickened by the clouds of incense. He swallowed miserably, his throat audibly clicking.

"Uh . . . I'm . . . *Steve,*" he said. Yeah. Another lie. They loved to lie about their names. I swear they thought that if they gave us their real names, they'd come home to rabbits boiling on their stoves and psychotic, knife-wielding strippers howling, *I won't be ignored!* But the key part of *Fatal Attraction* was the *attraction* part, and they never seemed to understand that actual attraction—of a stripper to a client—was beyond conjecture. In truth, they were as subhuman to us as we were to them: They were cash machines, and we were pussy machines. Customers could be *nice*—and by nice, we usually meant amiable and generous, without any unusually ugly erotic requests—but they were not our friends. Ever.

Girls who said their clients were their friends either were lying, or had such pathetically skewed boundaries they didn't realize how sad and preposterous their claims were. The nature of the adult business precluded friendship between clients and the girls they hired because friendship involves seeing the humanity in someone else, and letting them see your humanity, and neither of you telling lies to the other one. But the relationship between working girls and clients was *based* on lies, starting with our names and going on from there. Our jobs depended on covering any vestiges of our own humanity with a thick lacquer of fantasy.

Moreover, a stripper who considers her clients to be friends is putting herself in danger of being stalked, even killed. It happens. And the cops don't tend to wipe themselves out pursuing those cases. Most of them figure the risk goes with our jobs, and that if we weren't willing to assume that kind of risk, we'd get out of the business. And they have a point—jobs with built-in risk pay more, whether you're a firefighter or a dancer. If adult industry employment suddenly were to become regulated and safe, we'd probably be stuck making minimum wage all over again.

And worse than the pay cut would be working in a place like the Lusty Lady—a local, unionized peep show that hires dancers as employees instead of as independent contractors. Women at the Lusty are subject to a layer of middle management that dictates their appearances, performances, schedules, and wages. If a Lusty Lady dancer attempts to control any aspect of her own labor and comes into conflict with management, she's subject to punishment, or is simply fired. The Lusty Lady is the McDonald's of the adult industry, offering cheap eyefuls of pussy for large numbers of consumers who enjoy buying sexual service from women who can be fired for "unsatisfactory" work and who are powerless to dictate terms on their own behalves. The dancers make more than minimum wage, but the outrageous profits they generate for the corporation—instead of for themselves, as small-business-owning entrepreneurs—make them the equivalent, in my mind, of street workers turning their profits over to pimps.

No. Working girls have friends—*other* working girls. Customers are always customers. They have to be—it's the nature of the whole setup. If they wanted to be our *friends,* they wouldn't choose to be customers. They can have pretty much everything else they want on demand, simply by paying for it—but not real, human connection. They can't be friends *and* customers: They have to pick. And considering how much money's spent on the adult industry, it's clear that most men prefer being customers to being friends.

Mommy stared at me, frowning. I forced myself back on task, shaking my head briskly to disperse all my negative, nonhealing energy. I was here to get Steve's cash—that was the bottom line. The *only* line.

"Steve—I *love* that name!" I tucked my cheeks back, creating dimples. "Is that from Steven with a *v*, or Stephen with a *ph?*"

"Huh?"

Busted. *Jackass.* You had to have your backstory straight. The *v* or *ph* distinction was important for a name like Steve. I regularly created middle and last names for my noms de porn just so I'd never be caught in a transparent mistruth. Not taking that precaution was just sloppy, in my opinion. It marked him as an amateur. And that was good, because if he wasn't a fast thinker, he would be easy quarry. His false step was like the scent of blood in my nostrils—all of a sudden the chase was all that mattered. How much could I get from him, and how fast? Sometimes you could make your entire rent from one customer, if you managed him well. Maybe Steve was going to be the slot machine that paid off today, coming up three cherries and hemorrhaging quarters into my plastic casino cup.

Stripping is pretty much like having a compulsive gambling problem. The hope of the payoff always keeps you coming back, no matter how many times you play and lose to the house. Because we don't make an hourly wage or a salary, every shift we work is a game of chance: You could come in, get in costume and makeup, and sit there all day without doing any business at all. But when you're hot, you're hot—and a good hit keeps you coming back the next day, hoping to turn your one-shot success into a roll of good fortune.

"So is it *v*-Steven, or *ph*-Stephen, baby?" I asked again. It was a psych-out: If I rattled him, he'd be more likely to pay off. It was like tilting a pinball machine just enough.

"Oh! It's, uh, Steven. With a *v.*" He stared at the tantric poster on the wall in fearful fascination. Suddenly he reached into the front pocket of his Dockers, extracted a handful of pennies and nickels, and sprinkled them over the altar like a chef carefully adding salt to a dish.

Jackpot! We have the loosest slots in town!

For the first time, Steve turned and met my gaze.

"What happens next, Lily?"

I actually wasn't sure what the standard procedure was for taking a customer back to a practitioner room and getting him ready for his session. Lavender had handled that part with our eleven-thirty duo client, and I hadn't paid attention.

"Let's go into our room, baby," I said. Mommy's glare was interfering with my patter. Her silence was unnerving. It was like trying to act natural when you knew every word you said was being recorded.

Steve followed me down the hall to a practitioner room I hoped was empty. I didn't pick Lavender's, figuring she was probably hiding out in her own space. I fervently hoped he wouldn't ask to use the bathroom, because the last thing I wanted was to have to explain why the Temple had a six-hundred-pound barking woman stashed in its restroom.

I flung a door open—thankfully, no Lavender—and used the ambient light of the hallway to light as many candles as I could. Once the room was lit to the extent it could be, I closed the door firmly. Patting the massage table, I told Steve to sit down. He climbed up gingerly and sat there fully dressed, with his back artificially straight. Humiliatingly, his legs weren't long enough to reach the floor.

"All righty," I said. "Here's how this works. I know Mommy told you on the phone, but I'm gonna go over this with you again, just to make sure there isn't any confusion." *Smile,* I reminded myself. Abruptly, I grinned like a pumpkin at Steve, who looked frightened.

Good, I thought. His intimidation gave me a distinct advantage. Because I sure as fuck didn't know what I was doing—I'd never done this before, either. I was a professional-hand-job virgin—used to performing, but not to actually throwing down any real service. But after watching Princess Lavender do her session, I figured I could fake a decent show for Steve. Wasn't a hand job just a hand job, after all? Plus, after his initial terror, he might be so delighted at actually getting his dick touched that nothing else would matter.

"I'm gonna rub your chakras. All of them. At the end of the session you'll feel a *great sense of relief,* do you get me? And that relief is gonna happen on you, not on me. And it's gonna be when I say, got it?" I asked.

Steve nodded.

"Strip," I said. "I mean, *undress,* darling. I'm going to go freshen up, and I'll be right back in." I started toward the door, balancing on my toes like a show poodle.

"Lie on your tummy," I said as I let myself out into the hall.

Suddenly remembering a phrase I'd heard Mommy use on the phone, I stuck my head back into the practitioner room. I'd caught him in the middle of removing his pants. "Blessings to you!" I proclaimed loudly. Steve flinched, helpless with his Dockers loose around his hips. I slammed the door again.

Out in the hall, I took off my shirt and scarf, leaving my lingerie on. Baby stuck her head out of the bathroom and stared at me. "Miss Lily!" she stage-whispered. "Don't forget all seven chakras! Arf!"

"I won't, Baby," I said. But I was really only concerned about one of them.

I had to admit, this was heavy.

It was one thing to dance and model. It was something else to be fully illegal. And I didn't care how much this was supposed to be a temple and not a massage parlor, or how much legal immunity we actually gained from our stupid little fake-Indian word games and from making our customers pay afterward instead of before. I suspected that if a cop wanted to bust us, he could—all he'd have to do is say that I'd agreed to take money to touch his dick, and that was me with a prostitution strike, end of story.

But it wasn't the illegality that worried me. I was trying to think of the word for what was freaking me out. The only term that seemed at all close was *morality,* and that one was clunky and antique and seemed like the kind of word that only old people said.

And anyhow, *morality*—that was a joke, wasn't it? Because how was this any different from anything else I'd been doing for five years? I was closing a quarter-inch gap, that was all—going from one tiny little gradation of performance to the next one in an imperceptible flow toward . . . what?

I was scared. I was scared I'd touch Steve's dick and it would feel *wrong*. I didn't *know* it would, but I was worried that I would start and not be able to finish. For a moment I quailed, pressing myself against the wall. The wallpaper felt cool and comforting against my bare back. The wallpaper said, *It's not too late, you haven't done anything yet, you can still go* to my skin.

I could leave. Lavender could have Steve, and she'd kiss his ballsack and everyone would be happy. I'd never hear Baby's inane prattle ever again, or get barked at, or have to pretend that customers were *seekers* and that hand jobs were some kind of divine sacrament.

But wasn't *morality* something I had to figure out for myself? It wasn't something that could be dictated to me by leagues of disapproving old folks who used religious language to talk about something that was really about money, and power. Were those old folks going to pay my rent? If they cared so much, why did they try so hard to keep women like me miserable, scared, and powerless? Where were our options?

I suspected the people who liked to point fingers at strippers and call us *immoral* were pissed off not because they really thought of sex work as sin, but instead because adult employment removed us from their labor pool and allowed us to manage our own bodies and time.

Those old folks could wave their fingers around all they wanted, and try to tell me what was *moral* and what wasn't, but the bottom line was that they didn't give a shit about me, or Viva, or Nina, or Gigi, or any other woman who did what we had to do to make money without giving up our self-respect in this world, in the only ways we could. I loved those women with all my heart. They had shown me kindness and love and friendship, given me refuge—taught me how to work. They were good women—*moral* women.

So was I. Fuck anyone who tried to tell us we weren't.

Baby mugged at me, making her eyes bulge out comically as she waggled her tongue in my direction.

I ignored her, and slipped into my room to do what I'd come to do.

"Toxic" — Britney Spears

Steve lay facedown on the sheet-covered massage table, as I'd instructed. He was nude, though he'd chosen to leave his athletic socks on—a rakish touch. He'd found a clean, full-size towel and draped it over his own buttocks modestly, as if in preparation for a legitimate massage instead of a lackluster chakra alignment. I imagined whipping the towel off, twisting it, and snapping him with it brutally.

When he heard the door open, he craned his face toward me and stared, his mouth slightly open. "Are you wearing a wig?" he asked. "I was going to ask you about that in the lobby. It's okay if you are."

I was always amused by customers' attempts to reassure me that my appearance was acceptable to them.

Gee, really? You mean I'm pretty enough to touch your peeny? Oh, thank goodness I made the cut!

In reality, their opinions had nothing to do with my own sense of self-confidence. I had days I felt pretty gorgeous, and days I knew I looked like powdered ass mix, but after so long in the adult industry I had started to realize how little appearance really mattered. Making money was all about strategy. The smart girl got the money, with or without cellulite on her thighs or a towering mass of doll hair on her head. I wore a wig because taking it off at the end of the day created an even deeper rift between my work persona and my private self.

"Of course I'm not wearing a wig, silly," I said. I put the cock lotion into the Crock-Pot to heat, then lit a few more candles and three sticks of incense to punish Steve for his inquiry. I waved the incense over his body, fanning it toward his face until I was rewarded by a small series of gasping coughs. "Oh, sorry, baby," I said. I tucked the smoldering sticks into a small bowl of sand on the table, the way I'd seen Baby arrange the incense on the altar.

Wincingly, I checked the temperature of the lotion bottle in the Crock-Pot. I hated touching it—the plastic felt greasy, as if had never occurred to anyone to wipe it with a clean cloth after using it in a session. The lotion wasn't heated through yet, but it was slightly warmer than room temperature and that was going to have to be good enough. I shook the bottle hard and unceremoniously shot a phlegmy wad of lotion onto Steve's back. He stiffened—just like I had the day before under Baby's unexpected, infant-handed ministrations.

I relaxed into my work, kneading Steve's body like biscuit dough.

As I ran my hands over the knobs of Steve's spine, I imagined myself stabbing him in the back. For maximum damage I'd have to work the knife in between the bumps of his spinal column, prying them apart and attacking the meat underneath. A sturdy serrated hunting blade could be pulled back, tearing flesh on the backstroke, before being viciously shoved in again and twisted. I could almost feel his spinal cartilage popping under my fist as I slammed the knife home—could almost hear the whistle of his collapsing lungs.

I added more lotion to Steve's shoulders, digging my fingers in at the nape of his neck. He was so vulnerable, so exposed. He had to trust me. No wonder so many customers were frightened of us, giving us false names and paying us what we asked without question. We had unfettered access to their tenderest body parts.

If customers were honest with themselves, they'd have to admit that they looked at us—their fantasy girls—impersonally, as vehicles for sexual mileage. Some of the more reflective clients had to suspect us of looking back at them in the same spirit of matter-of-fact utility: Dehumanization went both ways. Customers want lavish, excellent service for as little money as possible, while we want to earn as much money as we can while providing only the most rudimentary service in return. In any adult transaction, both the customer and the working girl share identical senses of themselves as predators, and the other as prey.

I'd found that I tended to daydream about inflicting violence on my customers out of what I guessed was the same idle instinct that drove bored children to torture insects, pulling off their wings and burning them under magnifying glasses. It wasn't personal. Harboring a personal grudge would require seeing someone *as a person,* instead of as a thing.

And considering all the working girls who'd been killed or hurt by their customers, I wasn't surprised at my drift toward *Lustmord:* Maybe I was whistling in the dark, trying to shore up courage and power in fraught situations that could so easily turn dangerous.

I knew I wasn't the only working girl who had fantasies of killing or wounding her clients. Nina liked to terrify her clients by making her fingers into a gun and shooting them in the face while they came. She'd scream, "Bang, you're dead, motherfucker!" as they helplessly squeezed their own waste against her window. Gigi and I used to laugh until we cried imagining the customers' looks of horror and dismay—*shot in the face?* It never seemed to occur to them that they'd been aiming at Nina first.

"What are you thinking, Lily?"

Fuck you is what I'm thinking, Steve. Not for sale. Stabby stabby. I giggled. Since I'd relaxed, rubbing weenie lube into Steve's back had become almost fun, like finger painting. It was easy—all I had to do was smear lotion around and let my mind wander into various sociopathic, bloody little cul-de-sacs of my own invention. I was relieved to find that this part of the session, at least, was no big deal. I was in control, on top of things. It was nice to be running the session by myself, without interference from Lavender or anyone else.

And thinking about my friends made me feel strong and capable. We all did what we had to do, even if it involved touching warm cock lotion. I'd live through this.

"I was thinking about how hot you are, baby. I was just thinking about that big cock of yours, and how much I'm looking forward to touching it," I said.

I had a moment of intense anxiety when I realized I had verbally defaulted to *cock* instead of *root chakra. Pay more attention,* I scolded myself. If Steve had been a cop, my statement would have been undeniable grounds for arrest. But apparently, Steve was just a customer like any other.

"Oh," said Steve. He was silent while I worked on his upper arms. I amused myself by finger painting *dick* on his back, in lotion.

"What do you *really* do, Lily?" Steve asked, when I moved from his torso down to the backs of his calves.

"Huh?"

"I mean, what else do you do, when you're not here? Are you in school?"

Christ—a Relater.

A Relater was a customer who wasn't satisfied with getting the service he'd paid for as quickly and efficiently as possible— a Relater needed to believe he was actually *making a human connection,* that his provider actually liked him and found him charming. Men who use prostitutes and say things like *I made sure she came, too,* and *I only see girls who actually enjoy their work,* are Relaters. They are loathsome, and most working girls avoid them as much as they can afford to, because Relaters need to think they aren't, essentially, *customers.* They like to pretend they honestly respect the women who get them off for money. But their insistence on obtaining personal information from their providers is telling: They just want *more* intimacy for the same price, however they can wrangle it.

"Am I in school? No, baby. I'm not in school."

Steve pushed himself up onto his elbows. "Well, what do you do when you're not here?" He stared into my face, his eyes only occasionally flicking down to my tits, which were displayed tantalizingly in my padded black Wonderbra.

"Uh . . . I watch a lot of TV, I guess," I said. Wasn't it enough that I was rubbing the backs of his thighs with warm lotion? Did he really have to be a Relater? It was just my luck that my first solo Temple customer would want conversation as well as service. Chattiness was exactly what I'd come to the Temple to avoid. We weren't on a date. I was here to do my job, not to flirt over white wine spritzers and happy hour appetizers.

Shut up and let me do my job, cow, I mentally commanded him. *Stop trying to relate to me on a human level. We both know that's impossible. You're a cow, and I'm a milkmaid.*

Steve was silent for a long time. "That feels good," he said predictably, when I got to the big muscles of his ass. They all wanted their asses touched.

"Turn over," I said. Irritation was making me overly warm. I was sweating under my wig.

Steve flipped over and lay on his back. Nude, except for his tube socks. His body looked small and prepubescent. His penis curled against his body for safety, like a shrimp in a shredded nest of pubes.

He stared into my face. "You're beautiful," he said. "You're really beautiful." He sounded like he was convincing himself.

"Thanks, snookums," I said.

"Um . . ." *Fuck! Would he ever stop?* "Lily? I was just wondering?"

"Yeah, baby?" I squeezed the bottle of lotion over Steve's chest. The bottle made a wet, grunting noise as it farted out the lukewarm lotion. It sounded embarrassingly diarrheal. I hoped Steve didn't think I'd just cut one, or shat myself. But then again, maybe if he thought he'd annoyed me to the point that I'd lost bowel control, he'd quit pestering me. At least it hadn't sounded like a trumpet, or smelled like Chinese food.

"Lily? I have a serious question." Steve hesitated. "And if this is too painful to talk about, I totally understand."

Too painful? This whole limping conversation was painful.

"Were you, you know, *abused* as a child? Is that why you're here?" Steve stared into my eyes, his face and voice showing only sincere interest. But under that, I felt his greed, like a hand slithering up my skirt in a crowded commuter bus.

And that old chestnut—the sexually abused girl turning to sex work out of low self-esteem—I didn't know where that one came from. No matter how many stakes you shoved through its heart, it kept coming back. *Low* self-esteem? If I had low self-esteem, I'd still be working in a fucking coffee shop. It seemed to me that the gleeful focus on childhood sexual abuse in sex workers said more about most people's fantasies of what adult workers should be— hapless, helpless victims; damaged women—than it said about us. I'd known some working girls who were abused as children, but I'd known more who weren't. And who was to say that even if a girl was abused as a child, she couldn't make a rational decision about her adult employment?

That was it—it was time for punishment. I'd given him every chance to curtail himself. Now I was going to give him all the precious personal information he wanted so desperately—and then some.

Cow, you are about to be steak.

"Well, yes, Steve. I *was* abused," I said. "I don't remember much, but I remember that my mom and dad used to trade me around to their friends a lot. I was giving blow jobs before I learned to read."

Steve's eyes were round. "Oh my god," he said. "Really?" His cock twitched against the mat of his pubic hair as if it had been startled awake by the term *blow jobs*. He squirmed in pleasure at having made such a shrewd guess, and at having finally gotten me to speak in compound sentences about something both intimate and personal.

"Yeah, really," I said. "There are a lot of blank spaces in my memory. But I remember—no, this is going to sound crazy."

I shook wig hair into my face, bowing my head in shame.

"*What?* What do you remember?"

She likes me, she really likes me, I could see him thinking, *AND she was molested as a child!* Steve was in Relater Valhalla.

"Well . . . this sounds crazy, but I remember these *robes*— these long, black robes. My parents' friends used to wear them. And there were candles—tons of candles, everywhere. Like here," I said, gesturing to the flickering votives that surrounded us.

Steve shuddered.

"But you don't want to hear this, baby," I said. Fleetingly, I wondered what Lavender was up to. Maybe she was licking the mailman's scrotum, just to be sociable.

"*Robes?*" Steve's mouth made a moist little O. "Lily, is it possible . . . could what happened to you—could that have been some kind of *ritual abuse?* I mean, could it have been . . . *satanic?*" He licked his lips, which were rosy and slightly chapped. "What else? Do you remember?"

I bowed my head. "I remember—chanting." I paused. "There were some . . . animal sacrifices."

"Oh my god!" Steve's cock leapt and lurched crazily. It looked like he was dowsing for water without using his hands.

I spoke rapidly, allowing my voice to creep into a higher, more little-girlish register. "I was expected to fuck this one friend of my dad's? He was really old, and his breath stank really bad. He wore red robes, not the black ones?"

I lowered my voice to a whisper. "He used to fuck my mom, and I'd have to watch."

"Oh my god."

Steve was chomping on his own lips in uncontrollable excitement. I noticed with distaste that he had white flecks of spit in the corners of his mouth.

"I saw this on *20/20!*" he gasped. "It—there are *networks* of them, the Satanists! All over the country! The cops don't do anything about it, because most of them are involved in it too! And they just, the Satanists, they just pass their *own children* around. This is absolutely unbelievable—absolutely—"

Words failed him. *For once,* I thought. Too bad they hadn't failed him at the beginning of his session, instead of now when I was almost ready to prime his well. Still, though, the silence was nice. I'd finish him up and get him out.

Steve's prick was hard, standing rigidly against his own stomach. Without letting myself think about it, I squeezed a wiggly white line of lotion from his balls to the head of his cock. It looked like mustard on a ballpark frank.

"Yeah, it still freaks me out," I said. "Hey, Steve? I want you to *achieve release* now."

I couldn't think about what I was doing. I watched my hand move out through space and wrap around Steve's cock. *It's just another lotiony body part,* I told myself. His dick felt like a bicep—hard muscle beneath soft skin.

Now I'm a prostitute, I thought. *No, correction: Now I'm a satanic ritual abuse victim who is also a prostitute.*

I knew it wasn't funny, that this moment was actually huge and probably terrible and sad—or, at the very least, life-changing in probably about a thousand unforeseen ways. But I couldn't help laughing. The whole thing was demented. There had to have been some mistake: How the *fuck* had I ended up here, in this moment, doing what I was doing? Had my life up to now really led to here, to the Temple?

It was so unlikely. I hadn't been raised to do this, to *be* this. I'd gone to Catholic school, had braces, taken the presidential fitness test in gym. I'd been a National Merit Scholar. My life was supposed to have led from high school to college to graduate school in one smooth, uninterrupted arc. It was not supposed to have included a sojourn in the sex industry, or an extensive education in crass language and shockingly explicit physical performance.

And yet, here I was, at the Temple. I'd done my share of hand jobs for love, and out of curiosity, and for a slew of other reasons—some defensible, some utterly stupid—and now I was doing one for money, and I wasn't stopping. It was too late to stop. There was no point in not finishing.

I began to move my hand up and down. The lotion I'd put on Steve's dick decreased friction, allowing my hand to slide freely.

Steve bucked, snorting and whimpering. I was pretty sure he was imagining an old man in red robes having sex with multiple partners. Or maybe he was relishing the *deep, deep connection* he'd forged between us, that he'd discard and forget about the second he walked out of the Temple. Either way, I was nearly done.

"Steve?" I whispered. "*Come.*" I sped one hand up, and squeezed the base of his cock firmly with the other one. "I mean, *achieve release.* Now."

I pointed his dick toward his chest as he shot his load, which came out in several distinct phrases, as if separated by ellipses. As soon as he was done, I dropped his dick and seized a clean washcloth, which I used to remove the gross matter of his orgasm from my hands. When I'd wiped all that I could from my hands, I dropped the washcloth on his chest. "Here," I said. "You can use that to clean yourself up."

Steve stared up at me. "Thank you," he said.

I thought of Nina, with her flat chest and her hands in the shape of a gun. *Bang, you're dead, motherfucker!*

"You're welcome, baby," I said. "My pleasure."

It hadn't been terrible. I didn't feel too different, really. Mostly, I just wanted to wash my hands.

Steve dressed rapidly, then took out his wallet and counted out a series of twenty-dollar bills. "It's one thirty for the donation, right?" he said, avoiding my eyes.

But Steve, what about our deep connection? I wanted to wail. *I felt so close to you! Did none of that mean anything to you?* I imagined begging him for his phone number, and giggled.

But Relaters are just like any other customers—once they're done, you have to let them go as quickly as possible. Just because a Relater gets hard from coercing information from his provider and demanding that she respond to him as a trusted friend instead of a customer, it doesn't mean he wants any further interaction once he's blown his load. Relaters only want what they want on *their* terms, like every other adult industry consumer. He was done with me. Therefore it was time for me to disappear, to transform into a cloud of incense that he could wave away and disperse.

"Uh-huh, one hundred and thirty," I said.

He peeled off a few more twenties, slapping them down onto the table.

"There," he said. "I left a little something extra for a tip."

"Thanks," I said. Once he'd put his wallet back into his pocket, I escorted him out of our room and pointed the way through the main room of the Temple to the foyer.

"Bye, honey," I called after him as he reached the foyer and lunged for the front door. Steve ignored me and closed the front door behind himself decisively, as if trapping me inside the Temple—*where she belongs,* I imagined him thinking. A few moments later, I heard his car start, then the screech of his wheels as he pulled away from the curb.

When he was gone, I seized the money from the side table and counted it.

It was a hundred and sixty dollars. Forty to the house left me a profit of one hundred and twenty. For forty minutes' work comprising a backrub, a little storytelling, and a serviceable—if uninspired—hand job.

I could buy a lot of antibacterial soap and bleach with a hundred and twenty dollars. I could even afford to throw away my old wig and buy a nice new one.

Heck, if I kept working at the Temple, I could even afford counseling.

"It's Over Now"— The Automator

After a few weeks, I was informed that my picture—and my "healer statement"—needed to be posted to the Temple's website so that potential clients could look at me and determine if I was the *spiritual guide* they sought. I figured a lot of men were probably looking for a spiritual guide with large breasts, so on the day I was supposed to be photographed by Baby, I made sure to wear a bra with a few layers of extra padding and brighter makeup than usual.

I arrived for my shift and changed into my usual Temple apparel—a tight, long-sleeved shirt and an Indian scarf worn around my hips as a thin, easy-to-remove skirt. Mommy was quick to inform me that I needed to look "more like a healer," so Baby volunteered one of her massive saris, which wrapped around me several times and made me look lumpy and cylindrical, like a giant burrito. My breasts were completely covered by the sari material, and there was so much extra fabric around my middle that I looked waistless. Baby shot the picture from a low angle, making me look double-chinned and mountainous as I sat awkwardly in lotus position, my hands forced into stylized Indian gestures like those of the eight-armed statue on the altar. I protested to no avail, and the photograph went up on the website.

Predictably, my business dropped. Clients new to the local sex industry saw my picture and chose not to book with me, while customers who'd seen me at Eros Galaxy or Butterscotch's stayed away, presumably thinking that I'd let my appearance languish.

I did the best I could to encourage repeat business from the clients I did get. Once I had them in my practitioner room, I did my best to perform professionally, incorporating some dirty talk into my show and usually taking off my bra to give them their root chakra adjustments. Though I'd hoped to avoid pornographic language and poses, they were the only weapons I had. Despite the picture, I began to develop a small clientele, who came to understand that a session from me involved sexy lingerie, dirty talk, and very little time-wasting fake-Hindu "healing." I snuck a pair of high heels into my practitioner room and hid them, wearing them during my sessions and then shedding them before emerging into the hallway or the main room of the Temple.

Mommy grew suspicious as my call volume increased. "Lily, you're not doing any 'extras,' are you?" she asked me, her Mount Rushmore face stern and still.

"No, Mommy," I said. I really wasn't, unless you counted wearing high heels and moaning as "extras." By providing more visual and auditory stimulation, I was able to avoid more than the bare minimum of actual contact. My sessions were the exact inverse of Lavender's: She performed like a monkey on a stick, but naked and plain and mostly silent—whereas I told stories and flattered and teased and made sure to look as much like a standard adult fantasy girl as possible. It was annoying, but I was also accustomed to what I was doing. And making nearly $100 per session made it worth my while to continue.

I quickly came to consider Lavender's approach to her work as valid as my own. She was doing what she could to make her money, ultimately, and while I found what she was doing repellent, she clearly didn't. I guess if you didn't want to wear makeup or shave your pussy or wear scratchy lace lingerie, and you weren't smart or creative enough to embroider lavish erotic scenarios, the trade-off was ball-kissing, heavy skin-to-skin contact, and letting clients sniff your snatch. She had a right to run her sessions her way, the same way I had a right to run mine my way. And what had seemed like a shocking lack of solidarity with other sex workers—performing way too much service for way too little money—began to seem less egregious as I realized all the things customers wanted that she didn't, or couldn't, provide.

Eventually, as I met all the other practitioners, I came to realize that they were like Princess Lavender in that they really seemed to believe they were providing "healing" instead of just hand jobs dressed up with arrest-dodging frills. I had to wonder if they honestly believed that every customer coming to them—every *seeker*—was genuinely searching for spiritual enlightenment.

They were nice women—plain, un-made-up, and unpretentious—who looked more like yoga teachers than adult workers. There was a definite Temple aesthetic that I didn't fit into comfortably. In my wig, makeup, and lingerie, I looked like a drag queen next to my spare, neat coworkers.

After a few months at the Temple, I decided to place my own ad online, on a local bulletin board featuring conversation threads between local adult providers and curious customers, and "reviews" of various local women from clients, most of which tended to read like bad *Penthouse Forum* letters and included large amounts of wishful thinking. This had precedent—the other girls ran their own classified ads in *The Stranger's* Massage section, giving the Temple's number for all interested callers. Because we were independent contractors, we could do as much or as little self-promotion as we wanted. Smart girls ran ads as much as they could afford to: Many men preferred to believe they were dealing with independent providers instead of adult businesses, hoping an independent girl would offer bargain rates instead of hewing to the standard rates of a house.

My ad was succinct: I introduced myself as Lily, a new girl in town available for sessions at the Temple of Shakti. I gave a brief physical description and posted an old picture of myself that made me look sexy and marketable, displaying my shoulders and the tops of my breasts, though my actual nipples were covered modestly with my own hands. I included the Temple's phone number and asked callers to make appointments with my booker. I deliberately didn't include the Temple website's URL. The last thing I wanted to do was encourage an interested customer to see me looking like a formless mass in a clearly uncomfortable position, wrapped to my neck in fifty yards of bunchy fabric. I also provided my work email address, so potential customers could contact me with any general questions.

After my ad went up, I got a few dozen emails indicating interest and requesting more explicit pictures. I declined to send the pictures, instead emailing a short template thanking the potential clients for writing me and urging them to call for an appointment on the days I worked. There was a thin line between self-promotion and giving the appearance of being willing to perform outcall sessions, which were forbidden in any venue. I had no desire to see customers outside of the Temple, anyway—the idea of seeing a client one-on-one in an environment where I had no control and no backup, should he decide to attack me, was unappealing. The risk didn't seem worth the extra $40 I could make by pirating clients from the Temple.

When I arrived for my next shift, Mommy was in the kitchen, glowering characteristically as she stirred a bowl of Dinty Moore beef stew, which she covered with a paper towel and put back into the microwave.

"Do I have any appointments today, Mommy?" I asked. I liked to do two or three sessions per shift. I was getting used to the work, but the money still came as a welcome revelation.

Adjusting the customers' root chakras was still a deeply sickening act, but I swallowed my repulsion and did it. Their cocks seemed slimy and intestinal, like raw sausage in natural casing. I handled their dicks competently, using a hard, fast stroke even as they begged me to slow down, to "make it last longer." But I was merciless: My goal was to force them to come as quickly as I could. I tried to avoid as much contact with their seminal fluid as I could by pointing my customers' dicks at their own chests, letting them befoul themselves instead. One client shot himself in his own eye, then complained bitterly that it burned. After that, I aimed for their faces instead of their chests.

"Appointments?" Mommy checked her book. "Uh . . . looks like not."

That was strange. Since I'd posted my ad, I'd been getting at least a couple of sessions every time I worked. But the afternoon was young. A shift with no business whatsoever was rare.

The front door slammed open, and Baby burst into the main room of the Temple. Her cheeks were bright red, and she looked grim. In that moment I could clearly see the resemblance between her and her mother, especially in the small vertical lines that puckered Baby's forehead between her eyebrows. Her bindi rode the crests of her frown lines like a surfer breaching waves, waggling slightly but miraculously staying adhered to Baby's forehead.

Mommy had taught me to use eyelash glue to keep my bindi on. We all did that. At the end of our shifts, we'd peel our bindis off with our fingernails to reveal identical red spots underneath. We looked like cult members or zombies.

"Miss Lily, I need to talk to you," she heaved, attempting to catch her breath.

The microwave chirped and Mommy took out her bowl of stew, then stood at the counter spooning it into her mouth as she read *Woman's Day*.

Baby hefted herself onto the couch, forcibly exhaling with the effort of arranging her poundage into a sitting position. I waited, respectfully allowing her panting to subside.

"Sit down, Lily," she gasped, tucking a stray fold of sari under one massive slab of thigh. I squeezed in next to her. Our legs pressed together overfamiliarly, from hip to knee. I hadn't been this close to Baby since the day she'd trained me to align our seekers' chakras. Her limp, reddish curls smelled faintly of Suave strawberry shampoo.

"Lily," said Baby, once she'd managed to catch her breath. "I am very upset with you. Arf."

Her sad, singular bark made me feel deeply guilty. I wasn't sure what I'd done, but whatever it was, I pledged to apologize to Baby and do whatever I could to restore her good humor. I immediately pictured the high heels I'd hidden in my room, blushing in shame at being caught and chastised for such a hookerly transgression of the Temple's spiritual, healing atmosphere. A practitioner in heels was almost as bad as a practitioner saying *cock* instead of *root chakra*.

"Baby, what is it? What did I do?"

She frowned at me. Her bindi leapt. "You know what you did, Miss Lily," she said.

"No, I really don't, Baby," I said. "Please tell me." Had a client complained? With the exception of the man who'd caught an eyeful of his own semen—and that was hardly my fault, I hastened to assure myself—I couldn't think of anyone who had any grounds for dissatisfaction with me. I'd done what I was there to do in all cases—maybe too rapidly for the annoying customers who wanted me to lovingly tease, stroke, tickle, and entice them into orgasm instead of using force to extract their cock-snot with unrelenting military precision—but that was a matter of taste, and was easily defensible.

"I saw your ad," Baby said accusingly. "With your—breasts."

"Yes?" Was she concerned about my nudity? I'd made sure to use a picture that was much more modest than some of the other provider photos on the site.

"That picture made you look really—" Baby groped for words angrily. "Really *available!* Really—*professional!* Like a, uh . . ." She stared at me, her cheeks as red and white as peppermint buttons.

"Like a stripper?" I suggested. I felt a mild thrill of anger in my stomach. Was Baby, the six-hundred-pound procuress herself, actually accusing me of looking too *professionally available?* Where the *fuck* did she think we were? What did she think we were doing in those rooms, hearing confession and absolving our customers of sin?

"You looked, yes, like a—like a stripper," she conceded. It was clear that she actually meant *whore.* Her tiny nostrils quivered in offense.

"You didn't look like a healer at all! You looked . . ." Baby paused, winded. We both waited tensely as she struggled for breath. "I'm—I'm sorry," she wheezed. "I'm going to have to let you go."

I turned toward the kitchen counter. "Mommy—?" Surely Mommy wouldn't allow this to happen. She had to know that a girl who wore makeup and lingerie and brought in clients eager for dirty talk and high heels—even if Mommy didn't know about the high heels, I hoped desperately—infused large amounts of money into the Temple.

Mommy pointedly ignored us, scraping the bottom of her bowl with her spoon. The sound of her turning the page of her magazine seemed as loud and startling as sudden gunfire.

"Miss Lily, it's not just the picture," said Baby. "It's—well, it's your approach. You seem like you're in this for the money. And that's *fine,* it really is. I'm not making a judgment."

Slut, said Baby's eyes. They were pushed into the pads of her cheeks like raisins, making her look as if she were made of marzipan, or gingerbread. I imagined decorating her with ribbons of pink and white frosting.

"The other practitioners are here to heal," she said. "It seems like this is just a job to you."

Yeah, and when Lavender crawls on top of her clients because she's too stupid to think of anything they would be interested in hearing, she's healing them.

And all the ball-kissing, and earlobe-licking?

And the insistence that what we did here made us immune to sexually transmitted disease?

I thought of the Temple's stable of homely practitioners, each one as plain and wholesome as a loaf of whole wheat bread—not a tube of lipstick or a spritz of glittery body spray to be found among them. The full-coverage cotton panties. The unshaved body hair. The horrible *sincerity*.

I choked with suppressed laughter.

I was giving the wrong kind of hand job. And I was being fired for looking like the kind of girl men paid to touch their dicks.

I was flat busted, and Baby, Mommy, and I all knew it.

"I'll get my things," I said.

"Arf," said Baby regretfully. "I'm sorry, lovely Miss Lily. We just can't keep you here. I know you understand."

I did. I found it utterly ridiculous and hypocritical beyond human belief, but I did understand. When you looked at me next to the other girls, it was clear who didn't belong. Besides, I was using up all the antibacterial soap.

I padded down the hall to my room to retrieve my shoes. I didn't bother attempting to hide them when I came back to the main room of the Temple. Mommy and Baby noticed them dangling from my hand by their straps, and exchanged pointed glances with each other. *High-heeled shoes! It figures,* their expressions said.

Since I hadn't dressed for work yet, all I had to do was put my street shoes and coat back on. I donned them in the foyer, and let myself out.

I paused on the front porch. *So that was that,* I thought.

The irony of getting fired from a massage parlor for acting and looking like a massage parlor worker was not lost on me.

I trudged to the bus stop as the sky started spitting rain. I wasn't sure what I'd do next, but I had a little money saved, and time to figure it out.

Chapter 6
The Sacred
Feminine

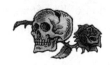

"Loco de Amor"— David Byrne

Goddesses wanted for healing touch, said the ad. It was in the Adult Help Wanted section of *The Stranger.* I quickly skipped to the end of the ad to make sure the telephone number given wasn't the Temple's. It wasn't.

It was a bad time to be looking for work, but I'd been eating Top Ramen for a week and scrounging through my pants pockets for bus fare. Rent was coming up in a few weeks, too. I figured I had a better chance of staying solvent if I kept my head down and stayed illegal for a few months. I didn't relish the idea of more touching for money, but it also didn't appall me. Going illegal was like losing your virginity: The first dick was the biggest hurdle. I'd already breached that boundary, so the idea of doing more of the same work didn't upset me much. I was more concerned about how sincere I'd have to pretend to be about being a *healer.* I'd learned from the Temple not to joke about that, even with the other practitioners.

I called the number and set up an appointment to meet with the owner of the business for an interview. We agreed to meet at a cocktail lounge near Northgate Mall at six that evening. In preparation for the meeting I did a load of laundry, washing my Indian scarf and my long-sleeved black shirt. I was hoping to start that evening if the interview worked out. I packed my wig, a few books, some makeup, and some CDs into my backpack along with my costume.

I arrived at six on the dot and went into the lounge. I wasn't sure who I was looking for, but when I saw two white women in saris, I knew it was them I'd come to see. I approached their table slowly. Interviewing for illicit labor was like doing a drug deal: You couldn't state your business or ask specific questions until everyone involved was satisfied that doing so wouldn't result in criminal charges.

One of the sari women was tall, her hair dyed a curious apricot color. The shade was somewhere between light orange and pink, like sherbet. I wondered if the color had been an attempt at strawberry blond. In any event, her hair was so fine and thin I could see her scalp underneath. She was in her forties, I estimated. Bad breasts, low and saggy. She wore a bindi on her forehead. She looked tired, but smiled sweetly as she recognized me from the brief description I'd given her over the phone earlier.

Her comrade was shorter—compact and dark, with a prodigious, jutting bosom. She observed me critically as I pulled out my chair and sat down.

"Hi," I said. "I'm Lily." I hadn't bothered to pick another name. Also, I figured some of the clients from the Temple might come see me at my new job, if they'd liked my sessions enough to remember my name. I wished Mommy and Baby no harm, but I wasn't above pirating a few customers from them to ease my transition into a new venue. A girl who brought her own clientele was welcomed pretty much anywhere.

"I'm Shiva," said the orange-haired lady, her voice high and tinkling, like tiny bells. "This is Devorah. We're *delighted* you could meet us on such short notice, Lily."

Devorah nodded curtly.

Cripes, I thought, *another good cop/bad cop massage-parlor tag team.* Was it municipal law that all Seattle hand job emporiums had to be managed by teams of two, with one partner friendly and the other one reserved and intimidating?

"So," said Shiva, quietly. "Do you have any experience in this kind of work?"

"Yes, ma'am," I said. "I was recently let go from the Temple of Shakti, I'm sorry to say."

They exchanged glances. "And why was that?" asked Devorah, in a surprisingly mild voice. I'd caught myself expecting Mommy's low rumble. She stared at me, the pupils of her green eyes pinned and keenly observant.

"Ah . . ." I didn't know what to say. I didn't want to trash the Temple—it was never a good idea to denigrate previous employers, no matter how loony they'd proven to be. "I, uh . . . I didn't fit in with the other practitioners, pretty much."

Devorah laughed. "You were probably too attractive for them, for one thing."

Surprised, I met her gaze.

"I don't know about that," I said, tactfully. I wasn't sure if this was a setup, a test to see how willing I was to disparage my ex-coworkers behind their backs. Nobody wanted to hire a girl who would come in and immediately create drama and dissension. "Everybody there was really nice. I think it was just that I didn't fit into the house very well—it was a small house, and the other girls had been there for much longer than me and they all knew each other really well. I was coming in brand-new," I said.

Warmed by Shiva's encouraging nodding, I decided to take a chance. "Plus, I came to the Temple from Eros Galaxy. So I was offering a more *fantasy-oriented,* uh, healing session."

Both women laughed heartily. "I'll bet that went over well," Devorah said, rolling her eyes.

"Listen," said Shiva. "I'll be straight with you, Lily. We need someone to replace Devorah, because she's taking a leave of absence for a few months." Devorah nodded. "She's busty and dark-haired, and so are you. You'd probably share the same clientele—if they liked her, they'd like you, and we don't have very many busty girls right now."

I inhaled and pushed my chest out. I wished I'd worn a padded bra.

"You're familiar with the work, if you worked at Temple of Shakti," continued Shiva. "I know Baby does a good job of training new workers. We've had a few girls from the Temple come to us, and I have no complaints about their sessions."

"Can you start tonight?" asked Devorah. "My feet are killing me, and I really just want to go home." I glanced downward and took in her spike-heeled boots. Clearly, these women weren't likely to be upset with me for wearing makeup and sexy clothes in my sessions. If Devorah worked in boots, I could work in my heels, no problem.

"I brought my costume," I said. "I was hoping I could start as soon as possible." I didn't have bus fare—I'd spent all my change on laundry, and on getting to the cocktail lounge for our meeting. If they hadn't let me work, I'd planned on spare-changing in front of the mall to get home. But if I got a session or two, I could take a taxi home instead. Things were looking up, definitely. Plus, I kind of liked them both—they seemed realer than Mommy and Baby, more likely to laugh and joke around. And Devorah's spiky boots were a clear indication that while they paid lip service to the whole *healing* thing, they were also realistic enough to know what most men were coming to them for. I was still going to be guarded, and outwardly respectful of all the spiritual stuff, but it was nice to know that I wouldn't be penalized for being a little dirty. After all, according to Baby, I was a *professionally available stripper*. And truthfully, I couldn't argue with her assessment: I needed to work someplace where I wouldn't be expected to be entirely honest with the customers. Devorah's boots told me I'd found the right venue.

"Great, Lily!" said Shiva. She dropped a twenty-dollar bill on the table to pay for their drinks without bothering to ask the waitress for their bill.

"Devorah, you can go home, sweetheart," Shiva said. "Lily, I'll take you over to the Academy of the Spirit and get you all set up to work tonight."

We stood. I shook Devorah's hand and thanked her for her time. She nodded at me, then left the lounge by herself, her sari flapping around her ankles. Her gait was awkward on the uneven pavement. I knew from experience that stiletto heels were really only reliable indoors, on smooth flooring. I wondered if she'd been a dancer before coming to work as a healer.

I put on my wool coat and picked up my backpack, then followed Shiva's pink, thinning hair out of the bar and across the street.

We approached a nail shop, lit up with a big neon sign advertising "Lotus Hand Silk Tips," a set for only $25. *Lotus hand* made me think of the horrible picture Baby had posted of me on the Temple's website. I hoped she'd taken it down the day she fired me. I never wanted to see myself looking so lumpish and miserable ever again.

Shiva slipped past the bright storefront of the nail salon and into a doorway that sat in shadows and looked as if it led to a basement or back room connected to the nail salon. The doorway led down a brief, dark alley, open to the sky. At the end of the alley was another door. This one had a small sign on it, saying THE ACADEMY OF THE SPIRIT. The *o* in *of* was filled in with a little yin-yang symbol, and there were swirly om characters around the borders of the sign.

At least it's not written in Magic Marker, I thought.

Shiva nodded at me, then opened the door. "It's always open," she said. "Just come right on in." I was pleased to notice that she left her shoes on as she stepped over the threshold.

We'd entered a living-roomish space featuring a kitchenette along one wall. Coffee was brewing in an industrial coffeemaker. It smelled good. I hoped I'd be offered a cup. Though, maybe the coffee was just for customers—I wouldn't ask for some until I knew if we, the practitioners, were allowed to have it.

Next to the counter that supported the coffee machine stood a large refrigerator, decorated with magnets holding up take-out menus, calendar pages, and photographs. The clutter on the fridge looked homelike and welcoming, like what you'd expect to see in the kitchen of a big communal household of students and artists. I felt even better about my decision to come to the Academy. The refrigerator at the Temple had been Mommy's domain, and nobody would have dared to deface it with magnets or cutout cartoons.

A desk faced the doorway, covered in an Indian shawl and bearing many flickering votive candles in little colored glass cups. Between two candles were business cards displayed in a carved wooden holder—*The Academy of the Spirit,* they said in fancy script, with *sacred feminine tantric therapy* printed underneath in smaller, plainer lettering. I assumed that sacred feminine tantric therapy was like chakra alignment, and guessed that it probably provided a similar *deep sense of relief.*

What was most immediately noticeable about the front room of the Academy was how many Indian-scarf-clad girls were milling in and out of it, constantly and rapidly. The girls coursed around us in a complicated circulatory system, too busy giggling and talking animatedly among themselves to take any notice of me, the new girl. The refrigerator was constantly being opened and rummaged through as girls selected food and walked out of the room munching contentedly, or swigging water out of bottles with their names written on them in black Sharpie. The front room of the Academy resembled an active sorority house's, except for the fact that everyone was dressed nearly identically in wrapped skirts made from folded squares of embroidered Indian cotton. It was like a cheery Jonestown, with individual water bottles instead of communal Kool-Aid.

I sniffed, sampling the air secretly. The Academy smelled good; it smelled safe and clean and welcoming. The coffee scent blended with the hot wax smell from the candles, and underneath it all was the good aroma of *girls,* and lots of them: makeup, scented soap, fruity body spray, and freshly shampooed hair, all blending together into one pleasing harmonious mass of fragrance. I could barely smell the stink of *customer* at all, though I was certain I would be able to sense the telltale stench of semen, fungal body odor, and lotion under the wholesome girl-smell if I really tried.

I felt a little overwhelmed, and too hot. I removed my coat and held it awkwardly, like an uncertain guest at a party.

"Ladies," said Shiva, in her clear, silvery voice. She clapped her hands twice. "This is Lily. She's new here. Please welcome her." The girls nearest me smiled, murmuring greetings. I felt shy and fought my inclination to hide behind Shiva's sari, forcing myself to make eye contact and to return the smiles and hellos.

"Fuck!" A tall, flat-chested girl appeared next to me. "Holiday!"

I gasped. *"Nina?"*

She was wearing a leopard-print sarong, I noticed, which hung from her hips saucily. Her hair looked longer—less severe, prettier and shaggier—even though only a short time had passed since I'd shared dressing room space with her at Eros Galaxy. We hugged.

"This is *my friend,"* Nina proclaimed. "She's *awesome.* Treat her nice." Her words implied menace, should anyone choose not to obey. Countless girls nodded, satisfied that I was known to someone they trusted. Like going to jail, being the new girl in any adult business was easier if you already knew someone on the inside. I was boundlessly grateful to Nina, both for being there and for claiming me as hers.

"Wonderful, Nina!" said Shiva. "Then I'll ask you to show Lily around. Do you have any appointments coming up?"

Nina checked the big black appointment book on the desk. It looked like the same thing dentists and doctors used to schedule their patients, and was covered in Wite-Out and scribbled handwritten notes in various colors of ink. "Nope," she said. "Not till eight."

"Great," said Shiva, smiling. "Thank you so much." She turned to me. "I'm so sorry, but I have to run. Welcome. Talk to tonight's phone girl, and she'll put you on our schedule." She kissed my forehead, lightly. "I'm glad you're here, Lily." She left in a swirl of sari and thin, pale orange hair, expertly shooing girls from her path.

"How the fuck are you, babe?" I whispered to Nina, as she steered me out of the main room toward a curtained-off, shadowy area I'd seen girls emerging from earlier.

"I'm good," she said. Something was different about her: Her eyes were clearer somehow, softer. She was smaller and less angular than I remembered her being. Of course, she was barefoot at the Academy, like most of the other girls who padded through the kitchenette gossiping and laughing. I remembered her in her towering heels, kicking the glass and lurching around Eros Galaxy in dizzying, ceaseless motion.

Suddenly I realized this Nina looked *calm*. Almost *happy*, if I had to characterize the nature of her tranquility. I'd never seen her at rest before—the Nina I knew was an electrical frenzy of rage and laughter and jagged energy, coolly robbing customers through the glass and then shooting them in the face with her fingers. This Nina was relaxed and watchful, taking everything in and responding with good humor. I thought of the word *gentle*. It wasn't a word I ever thought I'd use in reference to the Nina I'd known at Eros.

"Well, fancy meeting you here, bitch," she whispered in my ear.

We laughed. We'd both gone from legal work—even though what happened at Eros had very little to do with what was lawful, the work we did was technically called "dancing," and was open to the public and freely advertised—to *this,* the Academy. We were meeting each other a few notches down the totem pole of sex work. In a few short months we'd both slipped the bonds of legal (though shady) employment, and pursued labor that was frankly criminal. It was like running into your mom at the STD clinic, or encountering your priest at a swingers' club—all you could do was laugh and acknowledge that you'd both fallen.

I realized that Nina's contentment was due to her having found a place of refuge. The Academy was the opposite of Eros, a sanctuary instead of a battleground. She had staked her claim on a place here, a home among all these women. I felt a hard thrust of hope in my chest—if *she'd* found a haven here, with no Stewie and no horrible dirty plastic boxes and no urine smell and no cum-frosted glass, maybe I could too. The illegality of the work was a small price to pay for a place where we could earn money peacefully, without all the screaming and chicanery.

"How's Shiva to work for?" I asked.

"She's all right. We have our moments where we hate each other, and I get thrown off the schedule for a few days. She has her little freak-outs," Nina said. "You just have to let her yell at you. Don't say anything back—just let her go."

I couldn't imagine the old Nina letting anyone yell at her without exacting a swift and lurid revenge.

"Is she fair?" I thought of Mommy and Baby conspiring to wrap me in Baby's ugly, bulky sari for my website photo.

Nina shrugged. "Fair enough," she said. "She doesn't steal from us. And she lets us run our own sessions without trying to get into our business. She's got her own clients."

Score! The Academy was run by someone who did sessions herself. That meant a couple of things: First of all, she'd be physically unable to monitor us with any regularity because she'd be in and out of her room seeing customers. Secondly, as a practitioner, she would better understand the expediency of talking dirty and acting sexy for the customers. Doubtless she'd seen clients who'd wanted her to perform like a porn star, and whether she'd chosen to do that or not, she couldn't fault us for responding to their expectations according to our own comfort levels. Mommy and Baby had no idea what it was like to be in a room with a customer, so they had no empathy for their practitioners.

"Watch out for Shiva's regulars, though," said Nina. "She fucks them for the same price as a show, and they're used to that."

Bong. That was a problem—a big one. I stared at Nina in disappointment. "Fuck, really? Are you kidding?" I asked.

"Nuh-uh," she said. "Just be careful. They normally don't see anyone but her, but sometimes they try to see new girls to check out if they'll fuck for the same price too." She paused. "And if she gets a regular of yours, she'll generally ruin him. He'll come back to you wondering why he's been getting handies when he could have been getting laid."

Great. This was bad news—though upon reflection, it wasn't a deal-breaker. If Shiva had been prettier, I would have been more concerned. But she was older, and her weird pink hair was thin and sparse. Her tits were loose flaps of skin clearly unused to support from any kind of foundation garment, no matter how wirefree or unstructured. So some men would see her for mileage, but a lot of them would rather get jerked off by younger, hotter girls. It would even out. It was *gross,* but it wasn't inequitable.

"Do any of the other girls fuck?" I asked.

"Some do," said Nina dryly. "Most don't."

"Do you?"

"No," she said. We looked at each other.

Nina was marketable, especially with her hair grown out into soft waves. She was healthy, sexy, and a convincing performer—and what she lacked in cup size, she made up for with her long legs. She didn't need to offer any extra service beyond the standard house special, *sacred feminine tantric therapy.* I'd seen her with her heels hooked against the top of her window at Eros, spreading her labia and pretending to masturbate for legions of men feeding dollars into her booth. She had no reason to lie to me.

We'd gone past the curtain into the darkened back hallway. I looked around, astonished. The Academy was huge! A vast labyrinth of practitioner rooms and hallways led to still more rooms. Every open room I peeked into was painted a different color and had a slightly different design scheme. There were lots of Indian scarves and statues, like at the Temple, but there were also some Asian-inspired artifacts, like paper-lantern lamps and small, low tables. The place looked like it had been decorated by a crazy person who'd gone on a spending spree at Pier 1: Tatami mats and papasan chairs coexisted with brass Indian incense burners and Balinese wall hangings. Everywhere, votive candles and tea lights flickered.

"Holy shit," I said. "This place is *gigantic.*"

"This is the upstairs," said Nina. She led me down a hall—past more rooms—to a set of stairs. We descended to find still more hallways and rooms. It was dizzying. This place was Mount Everest: You'd need Sherpa guides to find your way out. I had a sudden desire to cling to Nina and beg her not to abandon me.

We turned a few corners, entered a large practitioner room, and from there slipped into a smaller, adjunct room. Nina flicked on the lights. "Ta-da," she said.

Against one wall was a tiny nest made of clothes and army blankets. Around the nest were several duffel bags and scores of books, some in milk crates and some in tall, unstable piles on the floor. There was a television set, its antennae decorated with ancient tin foil. A brand-new DVD player was wired to the TV carelessly, and dozens of DVDs—some with cases, and some without—were strewn over the worn carpet like rose petals. It was undeniably someone's living space. The room smelled faintly of cigarettes and vanilla perfume. I spied a pair of black patent leather knee-high boots tucked crazily between two piles of hardcover reference books. I remembered those boots from the peeps, and the smell of vanilla combined with Marlboros. I knew the room had to be Nina's.

"You *live* here?" I asked, amazed.

"Yeah, for now," she said, dropping onto her nest and slapping the space next to her. "Have a seat, Holiday. Wait, what? 'Lily'?"

I nodded. "I would have gotten shanked at the Temple for trying to keep the name Holiday," I said. "Way too strippery." I pictured Mommy advancing on me with her plastic fork held threateningly aloft, and the look in Baby's eyes when she'd said I looked *too professional.*

I looked around. "So, seriously, you live here? Does *everybody* live here?" I thought of the scores of girls upstairs, circling each other like kittens in continual, intimate orbit.

"No," said Nina. "I'm the only one who actually lives here now, I think. Another girl used to live here in the Academy too, but I'm pretty sure she moved out. And *I'm* moving out, too—next month. I'm trying to find a place near here."

"Dude, what happened to your old place?"

"A fire. I lost a lot of my shit. This is what was left." Nina shrugged as if to say, *What can you do?*

I thought, *No matter how much money we made at Eros, none of us bought renters' insurance.* An apartment fire had wiped Nina out. Now here she was, living in a jail-cell-sized room that was probably originally a walk-in closet, next to a room used for illegal activity. It was sobering.

"Shiva lets me stay here. I've been here since January," she said. "I work pretty much every day."

"You like it?" I wasn't sure if I meant the work or the room. Maybe I'd meant both.

"Yeah," she said. She smiled. "It's all right."

The Nina I'd known from the peeps was gone, dissolved into this sweeter, softer Nina. Whether her fury had burned away in the fire or had been tempered by leaving Eros, I couldn't tell.

We moved from her room into the adjacent practitioner room—this one was painted orange—and out into the downstairs hall. "There's a bathroom, if you want to get dressed," said Nina, pointing. I slipped in and changed into my costume and wig. "Will someone tell me if I get any appointments?" I called as I used eyelash glue to affix a bindi to my forehead. It was a little off-center, but it would do.

"Yeah," said Nina. "The phone girl books the appointment, then finds you and tells you what room you're in and what time your guy is coming. Tip her out at the end of the night—I normally flip her ten bucks per appointment."

Ten bucks per appointment, times how many girls? *The phone girl must be making a fortune,* I thought.

"How much do we get?" I asked.

"A one-hour session is one twenty. You keep ninety, and all tips," said Nina. "Drop thirty dollars to the house. You can give that to the phone girl and she'll write it up, or you can. I'll show you how."

Considering how niggardly most clients were, I imagined that the Academy got a lot of business based solely on the fact that a session here cost $10 less than the Temple. Plus, everyone knew what the girls looked like at the Temple. The ladies here—while still in ugly sarongs—were attractive and wore makeup. And I knew Nina wouldn't be caught dead looking as plain and washed-out as any of the Temple workers, or giving a limp, overly earnest performance. She was a pro, like me.

"Pour Some Sugar on Me"— Def Leppard

I finished getting ready by applying rosy lipstick, then did a final mirror check. I looked all right—busty and brunette, exactly the qualities for which I'd been hired.

I came out holding my backpack, my coat, and my boots, with my socks balled up together and shoved into one boot for easy recovery. "Is there much stealing?" I asked.

"Not too much," she said. "But it happens. Not as bad as at Eros."

I'd had my locker broken into countless times at Eros, and in one memorable instance, all my sex toys had been stolen. I was disgusted and amused to imagine someone so desperate for business that she'd steal—and use—another worker's dildos. I'd hoped that whoever snaked them had at least washed them. A few of them had been up my butt.

"You can put your stuff in my room, if you want," said Nina. "Or hide it in your practitioner room, under the table. There are a million places to stash your stuff here—just be sure to put it away out of sight, so nobody gets tempted. It's not so much the girls here as it is the customers. They're like fucking *magpies.*"

I shuddered, thinking of a customer rummaging through my bag in search of my underwear, or even worse, my ID. The last thing I wanted was for a client to know my real name, and where I lived. That kind of information leak could get a girl killed.

I left my stuff near Nina's tangled bed-nest, and we went back upstairs, where Nina checked the black appointment book on the desk. "Hey, you got one! It's for eight thirty, in the Blue Room. With 'Greg'; he says he's been in before but he's not a regular."

"Will you show me how to get my room set up for a session?" I asked.

"Yep," she said. "We've got a while before our sessions, though. Let's go hang out in the lounge." We went past the desk, through a set of glass French doors draped with the ever-present Indian scarves, and into a room furnished with battered couches and multiple space heaters, which buzzed and whirred and pumped out hot, stagnant air. Girls wrapped in blankets napped on the couches and the floor, while others applied makeup using hand mirrors. A few read, flipping through magazines or absorbed in books. Some chatted with each other, mindful of the sleeping girls.

"So seriously, Lily—how was the Temple?" Nina leaned forward, discreetly tightening our circle of two.

I glanced behind me. We appeared to be unmonitored.

"Those bitches were crazy," I said. "All of them. Holy Christ!" I described Baby's barking, and Princess Lavender's belief in her own invulnerability to disease.

Nina howled. "Oh my god, what the *fuck?* Does her mouth secrete 10 percent bleach solution? Is she, like, a bleach cobra?" She paused. "Oh, shit. Does she spritz her breath with Lysol before every show? Does she open her mouth and smell mountain fresh?"

"Dude, she did *research,* apparently," I said. "Maybe she was reading stuff from back when HIV was called GRIDS, and still thinks only gay dudes can catch it."

"Gay dudes? Half her customers would suck each other's cocks if they thought they could get away with it. And research!"

she scoffed. "Some customer told her to lick his nutsack once, and she did it for no extra money. That was her research right there!"

We tried to keep our giggling down.

At a little before eight o'clock, Nina got up, straightened her skirt, and presented a hand to pull me to a standing position. "My guy's coming at eight. I'll take you to your room and help you get it all set up. Mine's already good to go; I just need a few new candles."

We padded out of the lounge and passed through the curtain. A few feet down the hall Nina stopped in an open doorway, saying, "*Voi*-freakin'-*là.*"

The Blue Room. I went in, curious to see how a practitioner room at the Academy compared to the work space I was used to at the Temple. Right away I noticed the standard Crock-Pot, a pile of folded towels, one bottle each of lotion and oil, and various mismatched candleholders arranged like the study for a still life on a side table. Instead of a boom box, a CD-playing stereo hung on one wall, apparently wired to invisible speakers; the room hummed with ambient nature sounds. *Fancy,* I thought.

The walls of my room were a deep shade of almost-midnight blue, set off by white trim. Whoever had painted it hadn't bothered to mask off the molding with painter's tape. Splotches of white marred the dark blue paint all around the ceiling, giving the impression that pigeons had roosted in the room and released their droppings down the walls. Fussy lace curtains had been hastily thumbtacked around the room's one window. The glass, visible through the horrible curtains, had been painted black and was completely opaque. The lack of any light from outside made the room feel womblike and underwater.

Nina showed me where the extra tea lights were and placed a dozen fresh candles around my room, lighting them one by one.

Then she straightened the cotton sheet on my massage table. "The day girls keep the table in this room super low," she said. "You can mess around with it after your client, if you want."

I shrugged. I didn't care. It wasn't like I was a licensed massage practitioner, and it wasn't like "Greg" would be looking for deep tissue work or therapy for a sports injury—unless what he sought was relief for a pulled groin, in which case he'd come to the right sacred feminine tantric adjuster.

I laughed. I wasn't looking forward to jerking Greg's weenie—frankly, given my druthers, I'd be roasting it on a stick over a campfire—but lighting candles to create romantic ambience for some smelly, credulous clod who would be paying a little over $100 to use my palm as a pocket pussy struck me as utterly ridiculous. It was like serving your dog Kobe steak from a solid gold tray when you know all he really wants to do is tongue-bathe another mutt's asshole.

"You cool with everything?" asked Nina. "You need anything else?"

I couldn't think of anything.

"Oh, and the Purell's in the bathroom," she said. "I'll show you where we keep the extra soap and paper towels after my show."

Home.

One day, before my shift—after I'd been working at the Academy for about four months—I took advantage of the warm, bright weather to ride my bike to Golden Gardens Park. I pedaled along the shore and veered over to the dog run, where stay-at-home yuppie moms tossed tennis balls and Frisbees to their designer pooches while their babies waited patiently nearby in giant strollers. I parked my bike and watched the dogs race and jump for a while.

It occurred to me that I was well into my thirties, but I was still living like a teenager, sleeping on a mattress on the floor. I never felt freakish around other working girls because so many of us lived like carnies, moving from job to job and constantly hustling for new clients and new jobs and new angles. We were used to instability—feasting and buying exorbitant luxuries during times of plenty, and starving and hocking our costumes when business was bad. We traveled light, whether we were moving from city to city or simply from job to job, carrying our professional supplies with us and getting paid strictly in cash.

But as I stood there, looking at the women with their children at the park, I realized that other women my age had families, homes, and husbands. They were the normal ones, not me.

I had to be at the Academy at five, so I got back on my bike and headed toward the Ballard Locks. I was pedaling fast, trying to make good time, when a squirrel darted out in front of me and screeched to a halt in the middle of the bike lane. I clenched both handbrakes—skidded, for one endless, horrible moment—and went over sideways, breaking my fall to the pavement with the flat of my right hand. The squirrel observed me curiously, then strolled away, once it was clear that no squirrel treats had been dislodged from my pockets by my embarrassing wipeout. I was fine, but my poor palm was scraped and bleeding.

Damn it—I had to be at work! I couldn't have an open wound!

I used my T-shirt to brush the gravel out of the gash, then rode home, gingerly pinching the right handlebar of my bike with my fingertips to avoid painful pressure against my palm. By the time I got to my apartment my hand was on fire. The blood had scabbed over, but when I washed my hurt hand with antibacterial soap, the scab melted and I started bleeding again.

I called the Academy.

The Monday phone girl, Katie, picked up the phone, purring, "Hello. Academy."

"Katie, this is Lily. I fell off my bike," I said. "Do I have any appointments booked for tonight?"

"Oh, shit!" she said. "Are you okay?"

"Yeah, but if I don't have anything, I'm not coming in."

"Hang on," she said. I heard her turning a page in the scheduling book.

Please, please, I thought. I wanted the money—my cell phone bill had come, and I needed makeup that would cost over $50 at the M·A·C counter—but I couldn't work with broken skin. Even if I wore gloves in my sessions, just touching door handles and cleaning supplies would expose me to a host of infections.

"You still there, Lily?"

"Yeah. Anything?"

"Uh . . ." Katie sounded regretful. "You've got two. Do you want me to call them and try to book them with another girl? They both wanted busty."

Fuck!

Two sessions—that was nearly $200.

After a long moment of consideration, during which I struggled with my desire to stay home, to stay *clean,* I realized I had to go in. I had to make myself do it. It wasn't even about the money. I couldn't allow myself to turn down work in service of my own germ paranoia, because if I let myself start turning down work to assuage my OCD, where would I stop? It was a slippery slope that could only end with me unable to continue working in my field.

"No, honey, that's all right," I said. "I'll see you at five."

"You sure?"

"Yeah."

"Okay." Katie sounded relieved.

I didn't blame her. Calling customers and telling them the girl they'd chosen was unavailable was an unenviable job, requiring diplomacy and the ability to tactfully suggest other workers with similar attributes. Sometimes the jilted customers yelled, and sometimes they demanded to know where the girl was and why she wouldn't see them. Girls who canceled sessions a lot were major headaches for the phone girls. I looked at my hand. It felt buzzy, like bees were under my skin. Every so often I'd feel a slight sting, but it wasn't as painful as when I'd first gotten home and washed the scab off.

Sighing, I put on some makeup, being careful to use only the tips of my right fingers. *Just be careful tonight,* I told my reflection. *Bring lots of gloves.* I looked wan and unpretty, freaked out and tearful.

At least I was busty, though. That was something.

"Sir Psycho Sexy"—
Red Hot Chili Peppers

I reached the Academy a little before five and went down to Nina's room. She was out, so I changed in her room and hid my pack under some of her clothes.

Putting on my wig was difficult with only one good hand. I was squeamish about letting the hair fibers come in contact with my hurt palm because I hadn't washed that wig since I'd been fired from the Temple, and it smelled like incense and rancid head sweat. At least I'd thrown away the ratty, snarled old wig I'd worn at Eros. The one I currently sported was its replacement, and it still wasn't completely broken in, which gave me the giant-brainpan look common to girls with full heads of their own hair mashed under their hairpieces. The fake plastic "skin" where the wig fibers parted hovered a good two inches over my actual scalp, and lumps of my real hair packed unevenly underneath the wig made my head appear squashed and pulpy. Luckily, though, most men cared more about breasts and asses than they did about the possibility of their stripper suffering from encephalitis or craniofacial deformation. The bottom line seemed to be whether or not we were still, *technically,* fuckable. And even though I had a freakishly oversize head and one bloody claw-hand, I still boasted three theoretically useable holes. So I was good to go.

Once costumed, I tucked a Ziploc bag full of latex gloves into the top of my sarong, keeping it secure under the hip strap of my thong.

I went back upstairs and found Katie in the lounge. "Hey, girlie," I said.

"Lily! Let's see your hand!"

I showed her my palm. I felt like I was giving her some kind of Vulcan salute. She moaned sympathetically.

I shrugged, feeling like a noble, wounded hero. "It's nothing," I said. "Hey, who's my first guy? And when is he coming?"

We strolled out of the lounge to the front desk, where Katie checked the big black appointment book.

"Oh, you have Dr. Leon at six!" she said. "He normally sees Shiva."

Great. "Oh yeah?" I said, carefully. "Well, why'd he book with me then?"

Katie shrugged. "Shiva left a note saying be nice to him. He's one of her favorites, and he comes here all the time."

"Is he a tipper?" I asked. She shrugged again.

I was always uncomfortable waiting for my clients to arrive. There was always the possibility that they wouldn't show up, or that they'd show up and then decide that I wasn't what they'd had in mind for their session. I hated being looked at in my wig and sarong. It made me feel like a buffet line, as if my personal attributes were lukewarm steam table entrees on display under sneeze guards. *Pick only what you want, and have as much as you like!* Being evaluated for consumption by customers attempting to decide if I was appetizing enough to service them—my parts separated, cataloged, rated, and either accepted or discarded—made me feel about as sexy as a restaurant pan full of dry, crusted-over macaroni and cheese.

Dr. Leon was right on time. He was tall and deeply tanned, with silver hair and pitted acne scars on his cheeks. "Well *hello,* Lily!" he boomed. He looked me up and down, licking his lips. "I'm *very much* looking forward to our session," he said.

I disliked him immediately.

But then, I hated all my customers. Hatred wasn't a deal-breaker; it was business as usual. I didn't fool myself that my customers genuinely liked me any more than I genuinely liked them—we were there to do anonymous business as efficiently as possible, both of us vigilantly preserving our own best interests. Working girls were the equivalent of Jiffy Lube mechanics—service people, paid to perform a dirty job the customers preferred not to do themselves.

"Hi, baby," I said. "Wow, are you a real doctor?"

"I am," Dr. Leon said proudly.

"What's your field?"

He frowned. *Oops.*

"Never mind! What a silly question!" I giggled. It was never wise to ask questions that sounded too intelligent. I should have said *What kind?* not *What's your field?* The former sounded arch and cute, like I was asking what flavor of ice cream he liked best. *What's your field?* sounded like I knew what I was talking about.

"Family practice," Dr. Leon muttered.

"Gosh, I don't even know what that is!" I laughed. "Let's go to our room, sexy." I seized his hand and pulled him past the curtain into the dim hall.

In the hallway, Dr. Leon sighed. *What field?* had changed me from a hot, slutty dimwit—who might be easily tricked into performing extras—to a calculating professional who probably wouldn't give an inch without exacting a stiff toll. I'd gone from Pamela Anderson to Camille Paglia in one ill-considered off-the-cuff remark.

A girl I'd worked with ages ago at Butterscotch's padded by us silently on dirty bare feet, holding her Crock-Pot in both hands. She slipped into the bathroom and I heard her pouring the water out, then refilling it from the faucet. Her name at Butterscotch's had been Nadine, but she was Ariel here. She was a tiny goth girl who lived on Taco Time and stayed up all night, every night, dancing at a local vampire-friendly underground club. She spent most of her time at work in the lounge, sleeping or sobbing. The Academy customers inexplicably liked her—she always had at least a few appointments on the books. I wondered if her red-rimmed eyes and constant sniffling seemed exotic and adolescent to the middle-aged men who jerked off to their own moody teenage daughters and their daughters' black-clad, poetry-writing friends. Ariel always smelled good, like clove cigarettes and the rose oil she used in sessions with her clients.

Ariel emerged from the bathroom and paused, speaking to Dr. Leon in a low, sexy whisper. "Oh, you're doing a session with Lily? Lucky you. She's *so naughty.*"

"Don't make me come over there and spank you, you little brat," I tossed back. Ariel had seen Dr. Leon's pout of disappointment and was trying to help out with a little free girl-on-girl imagery.

Dr. Leon perked up. "Do you two . . . *know each other?*" he asked, his eyes darting back and forth between the two of us greedily. Clearly, he was imagining the two of us fucking each other, rubbing our nipples together and moaning. Men loved the idea of women playing with each other's tits and giving tiny, lizardy tongue-flicks to each other's crotches. They weren't so keen on the idea of us doing anything to each other that might actually result in orgasm, however. Lesbianism was foreplay, not the main event. Porn constantly reassured them that we needed cocks to come— real cocks, not dildos—and we blatantly reinforced that fallacy. There was never any money in telling a customer the truth.

"Oh, yeah," Ariel sighed. "You could say that." She giggled, then glided down the hall to her room, casting a flirtatious smile back at us over one bony shoulder.

Dr. Leon had visibly relaxed, my lobby faux pas forgotten. He was still licking his chops over the idea of me and Ariel getting it on— not to completion, mind you, but just enough. I hadn't gotten back to Pamela Anderson status yet, but at least I'd turned out to be a brazen, carpet-munching bisexual, and that counted for something.

One of the things I'd learned at Butterscotch's was that most men loved to fantasize about avoiding the need for foreplay. With their girlfriends and wives preliminary action was a necessary evil, but in the realm of pornographic fantasy, all that boring exposition could be dispensed with. Two girls doing each other fit the bill perfectly—it was the sexual equivalent of calling for pizza delivery and having your order appear, hot on your doorstep, in thirty minutes or less.

Ariel had worked at Butterscotch's long enough to have done her share of lesbian shows, though we'd never done one together. But she knew that the fast key to almost any customer's dick—the same key that unlocked his wallet—was the idea that his practitioner was all juiced up from girl-girl, and ready to seal the deal with the nearest available cock. Butterscotch's ladies helped each other out constantly, making shows of kissing each other on the cheek and flirting shamelessly with each other when one girl was saddled with a surly customer. I was immensely grateful to Ariel for her swift and adroit assistance—even though we were at the Academy and weren't as close as we could have been, she'd had my back.

I made a mental note to bring Ariel some Mexi-fries and hot sauce on our next shift together: I had her to thank for Dr. Leon's sudden tractability. I maneuvered him into our room easily, directing him to disrobe and find a comfortable position on his stomach on the massage table. I slipped out to thank Ariel, but she'd gone into her room and shut the door. I assumed she had a client and didn't disturb her. The hallway outside her room smelled of roses.

When I came back to my room, Dr. Leon was stretched facedown on the table, nude and nut-brown. His skin looked like a hundred cheap Mexican wallets, all stitched together. He was clearly a tanning bed habitué, and his tan line indicated that when he roasted himself under the UV lamps, he wore a tiny Speedo. Yuck. There was something gross and unapologetic about the kind of man who wore tight bikini briefs, reminding me of blow-dryers, Jimmy Buffett songs, thick gold chains nestled in mats of chest hair, and greasy rum drinks with umbrellas.

Reaching into the top of my sarong, I retrieved my plastic bag of gloves. I opened the Ziploc bag as quietly as I could and worked a glove over my right hand. The latex felt soft—almost velvety—from being pressed against the warmth of my bare hip. Once my wound was covered, I used that hand to squeeze warm lotion onto Dr. Leon's back, spreading it around with my left hand. I tried to do such a thorough job that he wouldn't notice he was only being massaged with one hand.

This was the part of the session I didn't mind, as long as my customers didn't try to touch me. It was finger painting to music. Peaceful.

I added more lotion and continued smearing it around. Dr. Leon's skin was so thick it barely absorbed any lotion at all. Massaging his back was like rubbing saddle soap into a leather jacket. It was all elbow grease—a tedious exercise in muscle. I doubted that he even felt my fingertips when I brushed them down his spine sensually. Subtlety was wasted on him—to get past his damaged hide, I'd need a jackhammer.

I usually kept my clothes on as long as I could, stripping down to my bra and G-string only when I turned the customers over, and removing my bra and panties only when absolutely necessary. The nice thing about the Academy was that the clients weren't there for a striptease, so I didn't have to shake my ass or prance around on high heels, tossing my mane like a show pony. I generally calibrated my performance to how needy or demanding the client appeared to be. A good client was one who lay on his belly with his eyes shut, flipped over when I told him to, and achieved orgasm rapidly, with no fireworks or moaning or repellent special requests.

If the customer seemed all revved up and wanted to get sexual right away, I sometimes capitulated and disrobed quicker than usual, but only if I thought he'd be satisfied with just that and not try to compel me to provide a longer or more intimate period of sensual touch afterward. Some of them wanted to skip the massage and spend the whole hour pawing me. I always demurred. I'd learned to say, "Let me make you feel good—you just relax," as mildly as I could, which actually meant *Settle the fuck down, Junior*. I tried to keep my voice mellow and nonoppositional. If they persisted, I'd tell them how much I enjoyed getting to know every inch of their bodies through sensuous massage and that by the time we decided to get a little naughtier, I'd be dripping wet and raring to go. Astoundingly and contrary to all evidence, most customers believed that they were sexually attractive, making my arousal plausible.

It was the pizza delivery theory all over again: If a customer could lie back and wait for the good part while a woman independently pursued what she needed in order to become turned on enough to fuck, or at least provide him some kind of sexual release, why not kick back and enjoy it—especially when she was being paid to do all the labor, anyway? I found that working *with* their lazy senses of entitlement instead of against them usually got challenging customers to back off, and let me do my job unmolested. The ones who just wouldn't stop diving for my pussy despite multiple *Let me make you feel goods* were informed that I was on my period and bleeding heavily. That usually stopped them cold.

There was no way I was getting paid enough to provide an hour of constant sexual contact. Not only was that disgusting to contemplate, it was a dangerous precedent—a customer who came in thinking he was "owed" activities of his own choosing was more likely to attempt to run the session, and a customer who tried to seize control of his time was more likely to become angry at a practitioner who didn't want to do something he'd ordered her to do.

So I usually spent at least forty minutes of each session moisturizing the client's skin with communal weenie lube, daydreaming, and listening to my music, curbing any attempts at participation by telling squirrelly customers to relax and let me focus on *them,* instead of myself. If they wanted to talk, I talked. I took care to sound painfully stupid, which most of them found charming. A few of them visibly relaxed when I deliberately pronounced words incorrectly or indulged in malapropisms, secure in the knowledge that at least they wouldn't be outsmarted. I talked like a baby, making my voice lisping and small to minimize my size. As a tall girl I had to be careful to give the impression that I could easily be overpowered, while constantly guarding my physical advantage.

It was time to flip Dr. Leon over. "Can you find a comfy spot on your back now?" I asked him, keeping my voice low and gentle. Startling clients who were relaxed generally meant starting all over again, trying to soothe them back into a calm and receptive state. They were like cranky babies, quick to fuss if frightened from a nap.

I held my breath, hoping Dr. Leon would turn without becoming agitated, or attempting to wrest control of the session away from me. Some customers were perfectly agreeable until the midpoint of their sessions, and then they got belligerent and started acting like looters in a riot, smashing and grabbing whatever they could. It was as if they realized their sessions were more than half over so they had nothing to gain by continuing to exhibit good behavior.

He grunted and rolled onto his back. I gave him a moment to reposition himself comfortably.

So far, so good. Go back to sleep, baby.

The room felt stuffy and hot, as if the tea lights had burned up most of our oxygen. I had to remind myself to breathe, and the air I got was thick and wet, like a warm washcloth. At least Dr. Leon didn't stink. So many other customers sweated out nasty, hormonal soups of funk when they got overheated or excited.

Suddenly I realized he was gawking at me. "What's *that?*" he said.

"What's what, baby?" I followed his gaze to my right hand. His silver hair bristled in oily whorls, and I noticed his neck was visibly ringed, like a tree. His skin was so roughened from tanning that it had cracked into hard orange plates, separated by tiny rills of raw pink skin. The thick chunks of hide overlapped in scales, creating a horny exoskeleton.

I shuddered. He was like an armadillo, or a dinosaur—there was something prehistoric about Dr. Leon's monstrous slabs of skin. A knife would bounce right off of his armor: my favorite in-session fantasy, summarily foiled. *How could a doctor tan like that?* It was horrendous and fascinating, like watching an oncologist chain-smoke or a gastroenterologist devour broken glass.

At least Dr. Leon's cock was soft and white, protected from the tanning beds by his jaunty mankini. I never thought I'd be grateful for a Speedo, but I definitely was in this case. His cock was living human tissue, unlike the irradiated layers of shale that covered the rest of his body. It hung off his lower belly in a sad little flesh-toned flap. I imagined myself saying, *This won't hurt a bit!* and ripping his dick off like a Band-Aid.

I took a deep breath, forcing myself to keep my voice even. "Oh," I said. "That's a latex glove, darling."

"Why are you wearing *that?*" he asked, his voice flat and disapproving.

It was time to change my glove anyway. I peeled it off carefully, exposing the scrape on my palm. I was Mr. Spock again, raising my hand in formal greeting and using logic.

"See?" I said. "I fell off my bike today, so I'm wearing a glove to protect us both." I chose not to elaborate. He was a doctor—certainly he'd understand. He probably wore them all day long himself.

I plucked another glove from my bag carefully and rolled it on, attempting a seductive nursey smile while doing so. Who knew? Maybe Dr. Speedo had a hard-on for one of the ladies he worked with. Either way, my *sacred femininity* was ready to get down to business.

"*What?*" he said. "Take that off."

"What? *No!*" I said. "Are you fucking nuts?" *Hadn't he seen my scrape?*

Dr. Leon sat up. "Are you for real? This is ridiculous," he snarled.

Whoa. Problems. I desperately regretted saying *fucking.* I'd been so stunned it had just fallen out of my mouth. I should have been more careful, should have had a better answer ready. Why couldn't I have just giggled, or said it was some kind of special sex glove, ribbed for his pleasure or something?

"Take it off," Dr. Leon said again. "I'm not paying for this kind of—*shitty* attitude."

My *fucking* had unlocked his *shitty*—great. Once a customer started swearing, things tended to get really dangerous really fast.

It was like swearing broke the social contract in which we both agreed to pretend to like each other and allowed us to view each other frankly, as despised adversaries. A customer who swears at you is a customer who no longer believes you to be someone who'll voluntarily provide him sexual release. At that point, you're lucky if he just leaves without paying. Some of them decide that if you won't do stuff willingly, they'll take what they can get from you anyway.

I had to decompress the situation immediately. Immediately as in *right fucking now.*

I quickly took off my shirt and sarong, then after a brief moment of consideration, unhooked my bra and stepped out of my panties. Tits and a smoothly shaven cunt were like shiny, jangly car keys to an infant—they almost always soothed a client who was becoming irate or hard to handle. A customer who was feeling ripped off thought he was getting something extra when his provider went fully nude, and all but the stupidest of them tended to settle down in hope of getting more special service for good behavior. I preened in front of Dr. Leon, desperately trying to reduce his hostility.

"Honey," I crooned. "There's no problem! I'm just looking out for your health, darling." Mentioning my own health was obviously immaterial to the good doctor, so I didn't bother.

"I can't get hard if you wear that thing," he said. He lay back down again, as if daring me to continue.

I took a deep, relieved breath. *He's lying down!* Maybe this would be salvageable—maybe I could act porny and moan and pretend to come, and by the time I went to touch him again he'd have either forgotten all about the glove, or he'd be so turned on I could jerk him off in a few strokes before he got a chance to start complaining again. I knew there was no way I was going to get tipped, but at least maybe we could get through the session without any more arguing about whether I had the right to cover an open wound on my palm or not. Smiling, I moved closer to the table, casually hiding my right hand behind my back and running my left hand down his chest. *Look, Doctor! No glove here, no way!*

Just when I thought everything was going to be cool, Dr. Leon reached out and roughly attempted to cram his fingers into my pussy.

I felt him scrabbling and scraping at my opening, as if I were a bag of chips he was trying to rip open. His nails tore me. *Weren't doctors supposed to keep their nails short?* I froze for a moment that seemed endless. I literally couldn't move—if I shifted at all, I was terrified that he would be able to force his fingers deep inside me.

Using the flat wedge of my left hand, I hit him as hard as I could. I was trying to break his fingers, but the angle was wrong, my blow clumsy and weak. Dr. Leon let his hand drop and didn't try to penetrate me again. He lay on the table, not looking at me, as if nothing had happened.

My cheeks burned.

This man had *patients?* This man was a doctor?

Anger curled around my stomach like a rat snake, cold and heavy. He'd expected me to obey him—to remove my glove and jeopardize my own health so that he could blow his load into my hurt hand. And when I'd told him that wasn't going to happen, he'd figured I owed him a finger-fuck. I'd already exhibited intolerable audacity in refusing his direct command about the glove, so he didn't even bother to ask my permission for the other thing—he just took it. He did it to punish me and to put me in my place—to remind me that I wasn't allowed to refuse *anything,* that he'd bought my body for an hour and I'd damn well let him use it however he liked. It all made sense if you divided all human beings into one of two categories: *worthy of respect* and *there to be used.*

Of course, he wore latex gloves with his patients. It was probably just working girls he found disposable.

I needed to get him out of my room. If I thought too much about what had just happened, I was going to kill him.

But, I thought, I'd kill *myself* before I'd allow him to not pay me, on the grounds that he hadn't received his *tantric therapy*. The only way to get him out was to finish the session.

"It's your choice, *Doctor,*" I said. "I'll touch your dick with a glove on. Or I won't touch it at all." *And if you try to grab me again, I'll kill you—I promise you that.*

My thighs shook in delayed reaction to his attempt at invasion. I clenched them together, hard. Everything had happened so fast— it was like my body was just figuring out what had happened. *Thanks a lot, survival instincts,* I thought bitterly. If he'd had a knife instead of just fingers, I would have been dead.

"Shiva never wears a glove," he muttered.

"What?" I stared at Dr. Leon, willing him to repeat himself. He didn't. He kept his eyes fixed straight ahead, avoiding my gaze.

I took a deep breath. "I don't care if Shiva fucks you without a condom, lover. And if that's the case, you'd better get your ass to the clinic for testing, because frankly, that little red blister on your cock looks a lot like herpes to me." My voice shook. I hated myself. He'd grabbed me and I hadn't even seen it coming. I'd hit him, and it hadn't even hurt.

"*Now.* If you want to get jerked off, I'll finish your session. If you touch me again—" I couldn't continue.

I realized that if I kept talking, I was going to start crying. Rage did that to me—I was a crier. I couldn't see—there was a black haze in front of my eyes that no amount of blinking could disperse. I'd heard of seeing red, but this wasn't red. Was I going to pass out? I felt his fingers against my pussy like they were still there. My crotch felt hot and infected, swarming with germs from Dr. Leon's filthy touch.

"Go ahead," said Dr. Leon. He still wouldn't look at me.

I approached the table, reached out, and seized his cock. I moved my hand up and down in absolute hatred, touching him roughly and not caring if my stroke was too rapid or too heavy. The hand job continued until Dr. Leon's soft white maggot of a cock stiffened, twitched, and then burped up a few drops of semen. I wiped my gloved hand on his stomach in utter loathing. Then I peeled off my glove, turned it inside out, and threw it into the plastic-bag-lined wastebasket as hard as I could. "Get dressed," I said.

Instead of excusing myself to give him privacy while he dressed, I stayed and watched him. Dr. Leon didn't like that. His cheeks were bright red under his tan. I thought of the Crayola color *burnt sienna*. He clipped a Rolex around his wrist, grimacing. Apparently the doctoring business had been good to him. He probably loved doing his female patients' yearly exams—liked feeling like he could go inside them, far up, and they couldn't do anything about it. I wondered if he pulled his glove off and pushed his fingers inside them that way.

Once he was dressed, he made as if to leave. "Put down your donation," I said. Dr. Leon hesitated, as if weighing the wisdom of arguing with me. I stared into his face.

Motherfucker, I will kill you. I will kill you and I will go to jail and it will be worth it.

My heart was pounding so hard I couldn't hear anything else. I thought of the Crock-Pot water. I could throw it in his face. I could use the ceramic pot to cave his head in like a moldy jack-o'-lantern, left out on the porch to spoil. It would be worth it. *Give me an excuse, Doctor.*

Finally, he took out his wallet and counted out six twenties. He tossed them onto the damp, twisted sheet covering the massage table. I left the money where it lay. Wrapping my Indian scarf around my torso like a bath towel, I opened the door and allowed Dr. Leon to escape. He walked out, keeping his eyes down.

I knew he wasn't ashamed of himself, though. Nothing that had happened had taught him anything about my humanity, or the personhood of any of the other women he paid for sexual compliance. My rage was pointless—meaningless. He wouldn't see me again, but he'd see legions of other girls. He'd pull the same shit with them that he'd pulled with me. He'd never know how close he'd come to being murdered.

I imagined I wasn't the first girl who'd wanted to kill him. I knew I wouldn't be the last. Maybe one of us would finally do it, someday.

Once he was gone I cleaned my room, mechanically stripping the massage table and gathering all the used towels and washcloths. I reminded myself to breathe. After a while, I stopped trembling. I'd used half a dozen gloves already. I'd have to be more careful during my next session.

I hadn't touched Dr. Leon's cock bare-handed, that was the important thing. I was still healthy—safe and sound. *You're okay, you're okay, you're okay*—the thought ran under my other thoughts like a banner of just-breaking news on CNN. Whatever happened—no matter how gross, no matter how ugly—I was okay.

Fuck him. I hoped he'd die in a car accident on the way home. *Please, God, please, take him.* Even if he didn't die in a wreck, his skin was so damaged he had to be hosting at least a few precancerous cells. Maybe they'd grow, metastasize. Maybe he'd die in excruciating pain, at the mercy of women like me being paid to change his soiled bedding. Maybe he'd piss off the wrong orderly, who would leave him nestled in his own waste until his skin bubbled with infection. The thought made me smile, hot and hard.

Once I was certain I wasn't going to cry, I dressed and went to the lounge, where I curled up in one corner of an unoccupied couch. I needed to be around girls. I couldn't *converse* yet, but it was enough to be in female company. I let the conversations occurring near my couch sweep over and around me, buoy me up, hold me tight. Something in me started to loosen. I breathed, releasing the physical symptoms of my panic slowly. I was safe.

"Hey," said Katie, looking up from her book. "How'd it go? That was fast." She smiled. She knew I loved shorting my customers on their time.

Breathe. I inhaled and exhaled deeply. "I don't ever want to see Dr. Leon again," I said.

"Oh my god, what happened?"

A few other girls nearby quieted, suddenly listening to us intently.

"He's a fucking pig. I will never see him again," I said. "Shiva can have him."

Katie looked scared. "Okay, Lily. I won't book him with you ever again." She came over, squatting next to my couch in her jeans, searching my face with her big, worried eyes.

"Are you okay? Do you need to go home?"

What happened? her eyes asked again. *Are you hurt?*

I thought about it. "I'm not hurt," I said slowly. "I'm okay. I don't want to go home."

After a while, the girls near us resumed their chatter. Katie went back to her couch, reluctantly opening her book to where she'd marked the page with her pencil, sending glances my way every now and again. She was checking on me. It wasn't unheard-of for a girl to say she was fine, then completely melt down. But I knew I just needed to sit on the couch soaking up the warmth from the space heaters, listening to the soft voices of my coworkers, and letting my bad session float away from me. I relaxed and rested my head against the threadbare arm of the couch.

I woke up when Nina bustled in, sexy and unfamiliar in tight pants and a slinky wife-beater and lots of smeary eye makeup, looking more like the hard Nina I'd known at Eros. She'd been out drinking with a boy she liked, and she looked beautiful and excited and was drunk enough to tell me all about her date, down to the smallest detail, and I loved it. I listened to her and I loved it and I loved her, and the lounge felt like home again, and I felt so peaceful and safe that Dr. Leon's attempt to assault me in revenge for not agreeing with him that I was worthless rose high into the air, eddying and swirling, to evanesce with Nina's cigarette smoke.

"Alibi" — Elvis Costello

A few days later I went in for a shift at the Academy and Shiva was waiting for me in the lounge. She was so upset her tiny pink nostrils quivered. Her weird, wet licks of superfine hair and her twitching nose made her look cute, like a baby bunny. When she saw me come through the French doors from the front room, her cheeks flushed pink in displeasure.

The shade oddly complemented her hair: She was uniformly rosy. I thought of Strawberry Shortcake, the doll that smelled like strawberry shampoo. The other girls looked up at me in concern—they didn't know what I'd done, but from their silence, I knew I was in big trouble. Dr. Leon must have told on me. Getting a complaint from a client was a major offense at the Academy and I dreaded the reprisal—but Shiva had never looked better.

Anger suited her, imbuing her with the vitality and forcefulness she usually lacked, with her tinkly voice and her serenity and her loose, low bosom. This Shiva looked almost hot. I could see this Shiva fucking a client, climbing right up onto the massage table with him, grabbing his dick, and riding him like a strawberry-scented demon. Then I thought of her fucking Dr. Leon, and it made me feel sick to my stomach. I expected she *had* fucked him—if he was her regular, it was certainly probable—and her anger meant she treated him like a VIP and expected other girls to do so as well.

She had even left a note for me on the scheduling book—that's how important Dr. Leon was. And I'd failed, antagonizing a major client. Now he was probably going to take his business to the Temple of Shakti and get his balls licked by a chakra-aligning healer for only $10 more.

"Lily, I need to see you," she said, her voice clear and cold.

I followed her to an empty practitioner room—the Red Room. Between Shiva's hair and her face and the reflection of the deep red walls, I felt like I was seeing in Red-o-Vision. Everything was on fire—dark and hot and angry—as if the two of us were trapped in a giant, throbbing womb.

I shuddered at the idea of seeing a customer in the Red Room—like waving a red cape at a bull, it seemed probable that doing a session in this room would only be asking for trouble. Because we worked in constant danger of customer assault, providing service in a room obviously designed to incite lust and rage was a needless risk.

I took a deep breath, inhaling the musty scent of unbrushed velvet and candle wax. So the room was blood red, dark, and scary. I was here to get yelled at and maybe fired by a hooker in a sari, not sacrificed to Satan on a stone altar. I thought of Steve the Relater at the Temple of Shakti. I wondered if he had come to realize that he'd been chumped—that the stories I'd fed him were all blatant lies, disrespectfully delivered straight to his face. Probably not—I'd been pretty convincing. A Relater like him was probably still jerking off over his memories of our *naked emotional intimacy.*

I put my head down. *Please stop laughing,* I begged myself. I tried coughing instead.

I knew I was giggling out of nervousness—I didn't want to be in trouble with Shiva for not accommodating Dr. Leon. I didn't want to be asked to leave the Academy. I'd made so many friends! I had my own water bottle in the refrigerator, with *Lily* written on it! I had my favorite practitioner rooms and could preempt newer girls from those rooms at will by placing sly requests with the phone girls and slipping them $5 or $10, the way Nina had taught me. I was part of the Academy—not one of the old girls, yet, but still: I felt comfortable and known. The Academy was as close to a home as I'd had in a long time: imperfect and sometimes chaotic, but those qualities just made it feel real. I had garrulous, loud, loving sisters and Shiva was our madcap mom, and the customers were just nasty people who came to our house every now and again to stink up the place and leave us money.

The thought of being a new girl somewhere else—in yet another fake-Indian massage parlor where I'd have to pick a new name and become accustomed to all the specific business procedures of a new house and learn whether they called it chakra alignment or tantric therapy or whatever else they could make up to explain why our hands were on the dicks of paying customers—made me feel exhausted and teary. The thought of being forced out of the Academy—forced away from the other girls, and from the warmth and solace of the lounge, and from the kitchen and the shared take-out food and the bare feet and the traded sarongs and the good smells and the laughter—that eliminated my giggling right there, like the big can of Raid in the commercials stopping all the cartoon roaches dead in their tracks.

"Lily," said Shiva. "Dr. Leon was very upset with your appointment."

I nodded. I wasn't surprised Dr. Leon had complained—it must have really shaken up his worldview when the dog he'd paid to perform tricks had actually stood up and refused his ill-treatment. I was supposed to bark on command, prance, balance biscuits on my nose, and jerk him off bare-handed. I wasn't supposed to spurn direct orders, or question his authority.

"What happened, Lily? He says you put on *gloves?*" Shiva's voice trembled. "Lily, he's a *doctor!*"

"I know that, Shiva," I said. I showed her my palm, which had almost healed but still looked a little red. "I'd fallen off my bike and hurt my hand that day. It was open—still bleeding."

We both stared at my hand, as if trying to decipher my fortune. I desperately wished my wound looked a little gorier. It looked like nothing, like maybe I'd just bumped it or something. I felt idiotic. "There was gravel in it," I said, helplessly.

I didn't know how else to explain my decision. It seemed self-evident that fluid-bonding with customers led to unacceptable risk of disease. If Shiva disagreed, nothing I could say in my own defense would make a difference. It was Princess Lavender and her amazing jar-sterilizing mouth all over again. I stared at Shiva in dismay. Didn't she want us, her practitioners, to be safe?

I was horrified by the suspicion that I was the only working girl in the world who didn't regularly allow my customers to expose me to their pathogens. Were condoms and gloves considered charmingly archaic, like hoopskirts or leeches? Was it like saying *thee* and *thou,* or wearing a bonnet, or Fletcherizing every mouthful at least one hundred times before swallowing? Was I a relic of a time when working ladies crossed their fingers, took their chances, and dropped dead of third-stage syphilis before reaching their twentieth birthdays?

I tried again. "Shiva, Dr. Leon wanted me to touch him with an open wound. I wasn't comfortable with that."

Comfortable—that might get through. *Comfortable* was like *boundaries*—both words were slung around by people paying lip service to the idea of self-knowledge and the power of healing intuition. Maybe Shiva would realize that I hadn't worn gloves to anger Dr. Leon, or to alienate him, or to give him poor service. I just hadn't been *comfortable* with his attempt to encroach upon my boundaries.

"Lily, he said you wouldn't let him touch you!"

I nodded again.

I couldn't deny any of the allegations. I *had* worn a glove. I *hadn't* let him touch me. Trying to give context would have only made me sound insane. *Shiva, he was disgusting and his skin was orange and he didn't like it when I wasn't dumb enough and he viewed my health as a ridiculous inconvenience and he tried to poke his fingers into me to hurt me.* How did I know that? Was I a mind reader? No matter how into alternative spirituality Shiva was, there was no way she'd believe that Dr. Leon had done what he'd done for the reasons I claimed.

If I told the truth I would just sound hysterical, like I'd had nothing more than a case of the heebie-jeebies, or some kind of free-floating "bad vibe," or worse, a *shitty attitude.* And if I got that way with one customer, what was to stop me from alienating other customers with my hostility? Speaking in my own defense would be even more condemning. I kept my mouth shut. Nodding—agreeing that I'd messed up, without attempting to offer any excuses—was safer.

"He was very, very upset," said Shiva. "Being rejected like that really hurt his feelings."

I couldn't help snorting. I suspected Dr. Leon's feelings were about as impervious as his thick armor of dead skin.

"Lily!"

"I'm sorry, Shiva," I said. "Will you please give me another chance?"

Shiva considered.

"I just don't know about the glove, Lily. What were you *thinking?"*

I stared at the carpet. There were globby, ground-in chunks of wax under my feet. I rubbed them in with my toes savagely. *Fuck you, Red Room.* Take that. I knew from Butterscotch's that the only way to get wax out of a carpet was to pick it out by hand. I wished Dr. Leon was on the massage table, and I was ripping his ball hair out with hardened wax. I'd make him watch as I put my gloves on first. Then I'd make him eat every last piece of hardened wax and hair. I'd make him chew every piece a hundred times, to aid digestion. Then I'd use my *gloves* to slap him hard in the face, back and forth, till he spat teeth.

I looked up and met Shiva's pink, rabbity gaze. She glared at me, her delicate features screwed down and distorted. This was the Shiva who fucked clients for no extra money because her tits were low and ugly and her scalp showed through her dry, orange sherbety hair. If this Shiva didn't understand why I used a glove to defend myself from Dr. Leon, it was probably because she didn't think her own health was worth protecting.

Did she fuck him without a condom? Because he was a doctor? Or just because he was a customer, and he told her to?

"This is serious business," she said. "I don't know if I can keep you."

"Yes ma'am, I understand," I said. I was nodding again. I forced myself to stop. The time for nodding was over—now it was up to Shiva to decide whether I was bringing in enough business to cover the loss of a major client like Dr. Leon. I thought I was, but I didn't do the books, so I couldn't know for sure. If Shiva thought I had a bad attitude or was intractable with clients, she might decide to let me go before I could offend any other regulars, no matter how many sessions I was doing. She had a business to run. The fact that she'd called a meeting with me instead of simply firing me when I walked in the door meant I already owed her a debt. Baby and Mommy would have canned me immediately for a similar transgression, I knew.

"I need to think about it," said Shiva. She looked slightly disappointed, as if she wanted more of an argument from me. But the thought of what I would be losing if I got fired made me too sad to fight. I wasn't mad at Shiva—that was the worst part. And I couldn't explain my actions any better than I already had.

I followed her out of the Red Room, padding after her silently.

"Shiva—" I stopped. I was almost afraid to ask. I was afraid of what Shiva's answer would be.

"May I work tonight? Or do you want me to go home?"

I thought of my empty pockets. I'd have to borrow change from Nina to ride the bus home. The thought of going home from the Academy empty-handed, in disgrace, made my heart clench like a fist.

All of a sudden my eyes felt heavy, and my vision blurred. The warm wetness on my cheeks made me realize I was crying. Not hard. I just didn't want to ride home on the bus by myself, with no money to buy dinner. I was lonely at home. I wanted to be in the lounge surrounded by my fellow working ladies, laughing and snacking and putting on makeup and exchanging stories, safe and snug next to my favorite space heater.

Shiva sighed. "I guess you can work tonight," she said. "But if I hear any more complaints . . ." Her voice trailed off. Neither of us really knew how to end the conversation.

"No ma'am, you won't hear any more complaints, I promise," I said. I wiped my eyes hard, with my knuckles.

That night was the first time I let a customer come on my tits. As he pushed his cock between my breasts, I looked down. His dick looked like a greasy little gopher head popping in and out of my cleavage. I made sure to press my tits together extra tight before the customer achieved orgasm, to make sure his waste would go on my skin, instead of into my face. The skin on my chest was intact, so it was yet another instance of *disgusting, but not technically dangerous.*

I wondered if in ten years I'd be bent over doggy style and taking it in the ass from a customer, telling myself that what I was doing wasn't technically dangerous. Who knew? Maybe in ten years, it wouldn't be. That would be good news for Shiva.

After the session, I wiped off with a blob of Purell on a paper towel, then slipped into the bathroom and washed over and over with antibacterial soap. I finished by slathering more Purell onto my chest. The fumes made my eyes water and my skin sting a little bit, but at least I felt clean.

I just didn't want any more complaints.

Chapter 7
On the Shake and Take

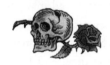

"Mr. Brownstone"— Guns N' Roses

I was sick of being cold all the time. Seattle's frigid, miserable weather crept into my bones and made me feel like I'd never be warm again. Even taking a super-hot shower was only a temporary solution—the cold was biting and permanent. I was sick of feeling clammy with chill all the time, and I was tired of the constant, horrible drizzle that spanned entire seasons.

More to the point, I was tired of working in Seattle. I'd been seeing the same local customers for years, and I was losing business to newer, fresher girls. I was at an awkward age by adult entertainment standards—not young enough for a "barely legal"-style schoolgirl persona, but not old enough to be viable as a wrinkly, saggy-titted "boomin' grandma" fetish model. An axiom of the industry was that if you wanted to make good money in your thirties you either had to start getting really nasty—like poor Houston, reportedly taking on six hundred men in a single afternoon in one legendary cinematic venture—or you had to be really skinny, really tan, and really blond, with giant inflated tit-bags, like pretty much every Vivid star over the age of twenty-five.

I'd been working in Seattle for seven years. I looked good but I wasn't brand-new anymore, and I had no intention of getting nasty or turning into a creepy, Nancy Reaganish, surgically enhanced pornbot. If I left town and went somewhere else, I could make a tidy sum being a fresh, mysterious new girl, unfamiliar to scores of local adult photographers and club managers. I could pretend to be inexperienced in the adult industry, and could shave five or seven years off my age. Customers—and most adult industry managers—love to hire providers who seem young and naive enough to be easily manipulated.

Also, I felt silly not taking advantage of the natural portability of my trade: All I needed were my costumes and shoes, and I could work anywhere in the world. I was a little ashamed of myself for never having left my hometown. I wanted adventure! I wanted to breeze into town, find a club, and work a few nights, then maybe stay or maybe move on to the next town. I wanted to be a cowboy, a maverick, a gunslinger! I wanted challenges, and yes, squalor! I wanted to have stories to tell my friends at home, and to make them jealous of my quick-witted wrangling in towns where all the adult service industry customs were different—where I would have to learn quickly, improvise, and rely on my own brisk intuition to profit. I was bored being a sullen, barefoot hooker in a sarong. I missed my heels. I missed glamour. I wanted a pole! I wanted to dance!

I'd been to New Orleans on vacation a few times, though I'd never worked there before. I loved the city's lush, wet, tropical heat. I wanted to feel warm all the way through again, to feel my muscles loosen and liquefy, to wear tank tops and let my ink show and breathe in as much of the hot, swampy air as I could. I wanted to sweat. I wanted to drink icy daiquiris and dawdle through the French Quarter and eat fried oysters. I was weary of Seattle's glum Scandinavian alcoholism and high suicide rate. I wanted to live in a place where people drank for fun or to celebrate something, not because they were cold and miserable.

I knew that New Orleans was world famous for its strip clubs. I knew I could find work there—and for the rest of my life, I'd have stories to tell about being a stage dancer on Bourbon Street. I was ready for it, hot for it. I wanted it so much it was like I *needed* it. Every time I thought of being onstage, looking sexy, and working the crowd in my high heels and work clothes, I felt a little tremor of excitement and glee that was almost erotic. I'd never stage danced before—so? I'd done everything else in the adult industry, from things that seemed benign and silly to things that made me sick, angry, and sad. I couldn't imagine anything that occurred in a public venue would shock me too much, considering my employment history. I felt like a boxer, bobbing and weaving, shouting taunts. *Bring it on, motherfucker! Bring it!*

I had a little money put away. I would stay at the Academy for another month or two to sock away a little more. I wouldn't need much to get started. As soon as I got there I knew I could find a job and would have cash coming in immediately.

I had to leave now, while I was at the top of my game, or I'd blink and seven more years would go by and all of a sudden I'd be an old warhorse, trudging along and adjusting my boundaries to reflect my decreased earning power. I'd turn into Shiva. And then in seven *more* years I'd be almost old enough to be a boomin' grandma, by industry standards, and I'd get a little burst of work lasting a few more years, maybe. And then my career would be done, and then for the rest of my life I'd feel ripped off and mad at myself for not having taken a chance on being the cowboy I'd always wanted to be. As much as I hated the idea of leaving my friends, the thought of growing old that way was intolerable.

I deliberately never allowed myself to think about what I'd do when I couldn't make my living in the adult industry anymore. Every time the thought of being old and without work crossed my mind, I resolved to save half of every dollar I made, to put it into mutual funds, to invest it and watch it grow, so I wouldn't end up a homeless old lady with no family and no work experience and no kids to take care of me. Of course, my savings plan usually only lasted until I saw a new pair of shoes or a work costume I really wanted. But a good wardrobe could radically increase my earning power, so wasn't adding to my costume kit just as good as investing in someone else's blue-chip funds? It was confusing. I hated thinking about the future! When it came, I'd figure something out. Just living from shift to shift in the present was tricky enough.

I was going to miss everyone from the Academy. I was even going to miss Shiva a little bit, though we'd never really recovered from our talk in the Red Room during which I'd cried and asked her to keep me on the schedule. After that night, it was like Shiva and I wanted to reconnect with each other—to get back to the initial peaceful boss-and-employee relationship we'd had when I started, half a year ago—but we weren't sure how to do it. So we avoided each other instead.

A week before I was scheduled to leave, I had my hair cut and dyed from black to blond. I figured that since I'd be looking for adult work in the South, being blond would give me an edge that might make up for my alarming amount of tattoos.

I'd decided not to wear a wig to work in New Orleans. Wigs were a hassle, and they always ended up smelling bad. Plus, wigs were *hot*. I couldn't imagine working in hundred-degree weather with my real hair mashed down under a big, glossy mane of fake hair. I'd sweat my makeup off in minutes and be lucky if I didn't end up passing out.

I wondered why I'd never thought to go blond before. It was actually very nasty. To raise funds for my one-way airplane ticket, I posted a picture of myself with my new hair on the Seattle adult services chat board. My business at the Academy noticeably increased. I didn't have to work as hard in session, either. It was as if my simply being blond was enough for most customers. I touched them automatically, going through my paces without bothering to talk much or get very creative, and I still made more on tips than I ever had before. The customers loved my soft blond hair so much, they were willing to overlook a host of flaws that up to that point, I'd taken pains to minimize.

I gave away my costumes that looked too goth or scary or punk rock, and bought some new ones at the Capitol Hill Value Village: white lacy slips, pretty pastel bras, and little '80s-style minidresses with giant polka dots or big black-and-white checkerboard patterns. With my chin-length blond bob and blue eyes, I looked wholesome for the first time in my life.

I threw out my heavy old red lipstick and replaced it with pink frosty lip gloss. I bought blue eye shadow for the first time since sixth grade. I looked like a loony cross between a Mormon girl and a porn star. My transformation was thrilling! I peered into mirrors and reflective store windows constantly, breathless and stunned. The new me was so beautiful, exciting, and full of possibility! I felt like I was pulling something off, something big, something that most people never had the courage to undertake. Discarding layers of my old self was like dumping ballast.

I didn't say goodbye to anyone at the Academy. I couldn't stand to. I knew if I tried I'd end up blubbering like a baby, and furthermore, if I said goodbye that meant I wasn't coming back. I preferred to believe that I'd meet my friends again, that I could come back to the lounge sometime in the future and seamlessly fit into the same old conversations. Until then I knew I'd be carrying every girl with me in my heart like photos in a wallet, and that I'd take them out and look at them and love them, and feel stronger for having them with me.

I wrote Shiva a note of resignation, which I tucked under her office door. I got on a plane for the Big Easy the next day.

"Start Me Up"— Rolling Stones

New Orleans was oven-hot, and so humid that walking through the French Quarter was like swimming in a pool that smelled of urine and vomit and bobbed with empty daiquiri cups. Bourbon Street was full of drunk tourists, even in the middle of the morning. I'd found a place to stay uptown, thanks to a New Orleans friend who had hooked me up with a friend of hers who needed a roommate. I had come to the Quarter to find work as a stage dancer in one of Bourbon Street's ubiquitous tit-and-ass emporiums.

The street smelled like hot garbage. It was kind of unbelievable how bad New Orleans smelled—like the produce Dumpster behind a grocery store. I was pretty sure the smell came from the garbage piles heaped on either side of the street, but a muddy, fishy element in the mix could only be coming from the Mississippi River. The resulting mélange of scent suggested a delicate blend of wino shit and dead rat.

That's because it's hot and wet here, like an armpit, I thought. *Everything is rotten, and rotting.* It was true: Even the buildings were tumbling down in slow motion. They were so ramshackle, it looked like you could put your fist through pretty much anything made of wood, brick, or plaster. Only the wrought-iron fences were crisp and definite, defining windows and balconies and serving as frames for hanging tropical plants or strings of Mardi Gras beads.

I walked down Bourbon, looking on both sides of the street for an eye-catching club. There were so many strip clubs, it was dizzying. I wanted to know about each and every one. I wondered which one offered the most illegal service, which one played the best music, which one had the hottest girls. It was exciting to see the names of the venues—Temptations, Scarlett's, Rick's Cabaret, the Sho-Bar—and try to figure out from the name and the look of the place what it would be like inside. It was also a little disheartening. I was brand-new to New Orleans, and I didn't know anything about the local adult trade. I knew I'd learn fast, but that wasn't the issue. I was conscious of being at a disadvantage—a new girl, in a new town. It was like starting all over again.

I was dripping sweat. My perspiration beaded up into pearl-size droplets and rolled from my face onto my T-shirt. Nobody else on the street appeared anything other than cool and serene. Tourists lounged in the heat with their plastic cups full of fruit-flavored booze, laughing—the girls in full, unmelted faces of makeup and cute little camisoles with skinny straps, and the guys in giant shorts and oversize layers of T-shirts. *Layers!* Maybe they couldn't smell the garbage, either. I felt the dull heat of resentment. Who *were* these dry, unruffled people? Didn't they realize how rude it was to look so comfortable, when someone who actually *lived* here was wet, sticky, and malodorous?

From the outside, Fancy's Foxhole looked just like the type of club I was looking for. I stood out front, staring up at its unlit sign. The sign showed a cartoon fox in a top hat and tuxedo jacket, sticking his tongue out lasciviously at a disembodied female leg that dangled temptingly in front of him. His eyes were little hearts. He clutched a fan of dollars in one paw. Over the fox-and-leg tableau, neon tubing spelled out FANCY'S FOXHOLE. The o's in

Foxhole had little irises and pupils painted in, as if someone were peeping through the letters themselves, curious about what was getting the cartoon fox so worked up.

A lot was going on with that sign—so much that I spent a long time deconstructing its various implications. Were we, the viewers, supposed to identify with the aroused, big-spending cartoon fox, or with the voyeur looking through the letters? It seemed clear to me that we weren't supposed to feel any sense of commonality with the single, seductive leg—even those of us who were approaching Fancy's to effectively *become* the leg. I decided I felt more like the eyes and less like the fox, given the choice—the fox was clearly a customer, a sucker, but the eyes were there to observe and discern. I felt a sense of gravity; if I got hired, this sign would become just as familiar to me as the buzzing neon sign at Butterscotch's that I'd plugged in at the beginning of every workday for six years.

I opened the door and let my eyes adjust to the gloom. I sniffed cautiously. Fancy's smelled like all dive bars everywhere: a combination of old yeast, hops, cigarettes, and hard alcohol—and under that, a thin, keen ribbon of bleach from the limp and dirty bartending rags used to wipe down the counter and clean glasses. The bar's interior was deep and narrow. I'd entered at one of the narrow ends, and I could see all the way back to the end of the club. A rudimentary bar was to my right. Past it a small, mirrored stage featured lurid red track lighting, with a bar and stools underneath. A brass pole occupied center stage. A velvet curtain led offstage to what I figured was the dressing room.

"Hello?" I asked, quietly. Where was everyone?

Seconds dragged by. I didn't know what to do, so I just stood by the bar. At least the air-conditioning was on. It was icy cold. I closed my eyes gratefully, breathing in the spilled-beer smell and willing the sweat on my face to hurry up and dry. I thought of the girls outside in their skinny-strapped camisoles, with their long, straight hair, skinny arms, and glowing skin. *That* was what I wanted to look like—cool, sexy, and unruffled.

"Hey—bartender'll be right with you," said a man appearing in the back of the club, emerging from a doorway marked with a green EXIT sign. He carried a plastic bucket full of ice. He came closer, ducked under the counter of the bar, and poured the ice into a metal trough. I guessed he was my age, or maybe a bit older. He had brown hair that curled in lazy loops and wore a plaid shirt with the sleeves cut off. Little white strings of fringe hung down onto his arms, which were tanned brown and dusted with freckles. He had a single tattoo on his bicep—a standard tattoo-shop black panther crawling down his arm, its claws drawing little red teardrops of blood. His gut strained at his shirt. The muscles in his arms and across his chest told me that he worked hard for his money—he had the big forearms of a blue-collar man used to lifting and carrying.

"Do you work here?" I said. Immediately I cursed myself. Of course he did—he was stocking the bar with ice. *Idiot.*

I tried again. "Is there someone here who hires dancers? I want to audition."

He straightened up from the ice bin and appraised me frankly. I tried smiling. He smiled back easily, then his eyes flicked down to my tattoos. "Damn," he said. "Did those hurt?"

"Yeah," I said. I always told the truth about that. I hated when people tried to pretend that tattooing didn't hurt. I'd earned every square inch, had shed blood and even a few tears for them.

I was coming to understand that by New Orleans standards, I was profoundly tattooed. In Seattle, my ink hadn't raised many eyebrows. But here, I was like an old-time carnival freak-show tattooed lady. I hoped that Fancy's was low enough on the Bourbon Street totem pole that its management would take a chance on hiring me. I knew I could make money—they'd see! If they didn't want me, I wasn't sure where else to go.

"Do you hire the dancers?" I asked.

"No," said the man. "You want Desire. She'll be back in two shakes. She's the bartender, but she's the one who hires, if we need anyone."

We stared at each other. "Well," he said. "I gotta get more ice." He turned, seizing the plastic bucket with one big hand, and made his way toward the green EXIT sign.

Suddenly he stopped and turned back to me. "I'm sorry," he said. "My name is Joey. I work the door here." He put down the bucket, scrubbed his hand on his thigh, and offered it to me.

"I'm Lily," I said. We shook. I saw no reason to give my real name. If they didn't check my ID, I could use Lily as my "real" name and then pick another name to work under—a pseudonym for my pseudonym. It was always wise to give out as little personal information as possible—a double layer of names would help keep my business private. It wasn't unheard-of for a coworker to accidentally reveal another dancer's real name to a client. Some dancers even leaked that information deliberately as an intimidation tactic, figuring that a girl who was frightened of her customers wouldn't be much competition. Most places asked for ID, and I always said I'd bring it in on my next shift, but I never did.

"Where you from, Lily?" Joey asked.

"Seattle," I said.

He laughed. "Nirvana, right?"

"You got it," I said. I wasn't sure how I felt about Joey. It was weird to be in an adult establishment talking to a man without hating his guts or angling for his wallet. Joey was a worker, though. I wasn't here to get his money, and he wasn't here to hurt me or trick me into providing extra service for no additional money. I realized suddenly that I had never worked side by side with a man, as equals, in any adult venue. Could I be real with him? Was he in the *friend* category? Could I trust him? Or was he yet another man to lie to and make fun of? If only there were other girls around, so I could take my cue from them.

I made up my mind to proceed cautiously. I sensed no malice in him. His face was open, and his eyes were clear, not sneaky or guilty. But you never knew.

"Hey, Joey, where you at?" cawed a voice from the back of the club.

"That's Desire. Hang on," Joey said. "Hey, Desire!" he bellowed.

"*What?* Come back here; Christ! You don't gotta yell!"

"You got a girl here, come all the way from Seattle. She's cute and she wants to work," he called back.

Cute. The thing was, I knew Joey wasn't attracted to me. He just wasn't—I felt no heat in his gaze at all. He was more interested in my tattoos than any other aspect of my appearance. He'd said I was cute out of politeness, to help me get an audition and then, hopefully, a job here.

Then he'd be my *coworker,* I reminded myself. Not a customer. Joey wasn't necessarily on my side, I knew, but he also wasn't *not* on my side. He'd given me a firm place to stand from which to launch my campaign for employment, a *cute* instead of a *no way,* a stamp of male approval that he could have easily withheld, letting me flounder for ground by myself. I was grateful to him for that.

A door slammed, and a tiny woman appeared, a cigarette bristling from her mouth. She strode out, swinging her hips proudly like a toreador. She was shaped like a beer keg, with a high, round, waistless torso propped up on short, skinny legs. Her arms looked as slender as pins next to her stocky middle. From the drumlike tightness of her belly, I guessed her bloat came from alcohol. Female fat was usually soft, particularly belly fat; a hard, swollen gut like Desire's usually only developed as a result of years of heavy drinking, I'd found. I'd worked with a few long-term alcoholics, and I was always amazed at how unaffected and smooth their limbs were in comparison to their puffy, exhausted faces and distended middles.

Desire puffed on her smoke and took me in. Her eyes swept from my hair to my shoes, then back up again. She stared into my face challengingly, drawing so hard on her cigarette her mouth looked seamed, as if it had been stitched shut. I tried to look sweet and uncomplicated.

"You got some tattoos, girl," she said slowly.

"Yes ma'am, I do," I said. I changed the subject as tactfully as I could. "I just got here from Seattle. I'm looking for work."

Joey picked up the plastic bucket and hurried toward the green EXIT sign, moving quickly under Desire's sudden scrutiny. "Get me some Heineken," she said. "Two of them." *Two uh dem.*

Her accent was almost Brooklyny, but I knew it belonged here. I'd heard the same accent from other New Orleanians, and I'd read about it in books like John Kennedy Toole's *Confederacy of Dunces*. It was thrilling and alien. Nobody in Seattle talked like that, ever—unless they were pretending to be East Coast wiseguys, saying *dese* and *dose* instead of *these* and *those*. I managed to restrain myself from asking her to repeat herself so I could hear her say *dem* again.

I was so far from home. Two weeks ago I'd been working at the Academy, surrounded by friends. Now here I was in this swampy town, all by myself. Regardless of whether I failed or triumphed in this bar, I'd have nobody to talk to after it was over.

The few friends of mine who had never danced didn't understand any of the challenges—they just thought I got up, danced around, and collected money from men who were so grateful to bask in my beauty that they couldn't wait to pay me anything I asked. They also assumed I did adult work because I loved being looked at, and showing off, and being "sexy." They didn't realize there was nothing sexy about adult work—that it was just a customer service job, much like any other. The only eroticism generated by stripping was all on the customers' end, occurring in their heads as they watched real girls dance around like puppets in front of them. Being stared at was mostly neutral, intermittently fun, and sometimes horrible. It was part of the job, that was all. I was pretty shy in real life, and I didn't like wearing flashy clothes or dressing immodestly. I was about as far from an exhibitionist as you could get. The notion that I stripped for any other reason than an economic one was utterly ridiculous.

Desire puffed on her cigarette. "You got your stuff to audition?"

"Yeah!" I said. *Holy shit*—I had a chance. That was all I needed.

I could do this. I could totally do this. Once Desire saw me in my costume, she'd forget about my tattoos and I'd have a job, I knew I would. I was a professional. Just because I was in a city that smelled like garbage, where people said *dem* and shamelessly consumed hard liquor on the street, that didn't mean I couldn't do the same thing here that I'd been doing for years in the Northwest. Tits were tits and ass was ass, and that was the bottom line.

"The dressing room's back there," said Desire. "Under the EXIT sign, to the right. So's the jukebox. Just look through the songs and tell me what you want to play." She stubbed out her smoke in one of the plastic ashtrays arranged every few feet along the length of the bar. "You nervous?" she said, eyeing me.

"Nah," I said. I didn't know if I was or not. I *had* been, a few moments before, but now, I just wanted to get changed and get onstage. I was a boxer, slipping in my mouth guard and climbing into the ring. All I needed to hear was the bell, and I'd come out swinging. *Two hits, baby—me hitting you, and you hitting the floor.* I laughed.

"Thanks," I said, and went back into the club, past the EXIT sign, and to the right, the way Desire had instructed.

"So Alive"— Love and Rockets

I found myself in a tiny dressing room. Lockers held up one wall. A long mirror with a counter underneath faced the lockers. Standard. *Fuck This Shit* was written in black Sharpie on the crumbling plaster wall, over the mirror. The phrase was surrounded by little puffy hearts, interspersed with dollar signs and stars. In the corner was a jukebox, the cracked plastic faceplate patched and held to the body of the machine with strips of black duct tape. Some of the lockers hung open, as if they'd been pried open and abandoned. An ancient G-string was cavalierly thumbtacked to the wall. Someone had drawn an arrow on the wall pointing to the panties, without bothering to leave any other written comment or explanation.

I dropped my backpack on the floor, pulled it open, and changed quickly. Once I was in my bra, thong, stockings, and slip, I redid my makeup, adding as much powder as I could to take the shine off my face. I licked my index fingers and used them to clean the makeup from under my eyes. Then I added more black eye pencil and finished with a coat of pink lip gloss. I looked all right— at least you could see that I actually had a waist, which had up to that point been hidden under my damp, stretched-out T-shirt. I still wasn't used to seeing myself with my blond Little Dutch Boy hair. I pulled on long satin gloves, to cover most of my ink. On the whole, I was pretty pleased with the results. I'd gone from chunky metal babe to viable stripper in about seven minutes.

271

I slid on my heels and lurched over to the jukebox. I was disappointed to see that most of my choices were either R&B, rap, or Top 40 alternative stuff that was impossible to dance to, in my opinion. I was looking for old metal or something with a slow, nasty grind to it. The pickings were slim, but I eventually picked out two songs, memorizing the letter and number next to each one.

I emerged from the dressing room and went back to the bar, where Desire was smoking and moodily paging through a *Family Circle*. When she heard me coming, she put the magazine down and watched me approach. I tried not to stagger but the carpet was all rucked up and uneven, as if the carpet pad underneath had dissolved or been eaten away in spots. It was easier to walk if I shifted all my weight forward and tiptoed. I minced over to Desire like the world's chubbiest ballerina.

"You look nice," Desire said. "That's an improvement."

I smiled. I was pretty sure she hadn't meant to be insulting.

"How many songs do you want me to do?" I asked.

"One is fine," she said. "I'll probably stop you somewhere in the middle." She took a long, speculative drag on her cigarette. "Hey! *Joey!*"

Joey stuck his head out from the back. "Yes, ma'am?"

Desire poured a shot of Jack Daniels into a plastic shot glass, which she set on the bar decisively. "Come on over here, babe. Take this and be a customer." *Take dis'n be a customah.*

I felt like a girl in a movie. I was going to audition for a Bourbon Street strip club. Even if it was Fancy's Foxhole instead of *Hustler,* I was still impressed with my own fearlessness. I didn't think about what would happen if I didn't pass the audition. I had about $75 left, tucked into my boot in the little room I'd rented uptown—not enough to get me home to Seattle, not by far. I needed work badly.

Joey retrieved his shot and sat on a high stool covered in ripped red plastic in front of the stage, dead center. He didn't look at me. He hunched over, as if protecting his plastic shot glass from imaginary people on either side of him.

"Hey! Hey, uh—what's your name?" Desire lit another cigarette, holding it between her teeth precisely, revealing a smudge of coral lipstick across her front teeth and gums.

"It's, uh . . ." I hadn't thought of what name I wanted to use. *Fuck.* I was going to be Lily again. I was getting very, very sick of that name. "It's Lily," I said. I figured I could always change it later. Girls did that all the time.

"Okay, Lily—what song you want, babe?"

"55-C," I said. "Hey, is this city down to topless, or fully nude?"

"Topless only. Keep your G-string on, *always*," said Desire, archly. "No touching yourself. No nasty stuff onstage."

"Can I spank myself and touch my own boobs?" I felt like a compulsive masturbator asking that, but I had to know. It made a huge difference in the quality of my routine.

"Yeah," she said. "But don't, you know, *play* with your boobies like you're gonna get off. You gotta save that for your private shows. Spanking's okay—go for it if you want. No messin' around in your panties, though."

I nodded. Easy-peasy. I was relieved at not having to take my G-string off. I'd never been good at taking my panties off over my shoes from a standing position, and when I took them off lying down, they always seemed to catch on my ankle strap. *No messin' around in your panties* meant no fake masturbation, which was fabulous. I was sick of rubbing the front of my thong and moaning. I'd already made a career out of that at Butterscotch's, and the thought of doing it here—in front of Joey now, and a club full of completely clothed men later—was tedious and unappealing.

"All righty, go on up. I'll put your song on for you." Desire carefully parked her cigarette in an ashtray, leaving it to smolder like incense.

I walked past Joey—who still wouldn't look at me. I was still walking like I was neurologically impaired. I could only hope the wooden stage would be friendlier to my shoes. If it was as craterous as the carpet, I'd get down and do a floor routine. I had a fairly good repertoire of floor poses I'd developed over the years to camouflage my height. Most short men didn't want their stripper to tower over them, and I was a few inches over six feet tall in my heels.

When the first few notes of my song came on, I took a deep breath, climbed the stairs, and moved the curtain aside. No problem. This was nothing. I looked damn good and that was all that mattered. Even if I didn't look that great, I had big tits, all jacked up in my padded push-up bra. And even if my tits weren't that big, I could smile and look like I was having the time of my life. I knew I could do that, for a fact.

I'd picked "Back in Black," by AC/DC. It was a little faster than I was used to, but I wanted something fairly aggressive that would do a lot of my work for me while I got my bearings. I pushed the velvet curtain aside, and sauntered out onto the stage, my heart pounding.

The secret to stripping when you're nervous, sick, or exhausted is this: Move super slow—*not* to the beat. Even if you just stand there, look confident. Move your hand to your hip, then shift your weight to that hip. Smile like you're making fun of the whole "I'm stripping for you" thing—like it's just silly and you're in on the joke. The customers will love you for barely trying, much more than they'd love you if you were earnest.

I figured that if men wanted to see a girl actually *dance,* they'd go to the ballet. In a strip club they're there to fantasize, and the best grist for their imagination is a projection of pluck and personality. They want to think, *Oh, that girl looks like a real good time,* not *Wow, that girl can really pirouette.*

I started against the mirror, with my back to my lone, slumped *customah*. I reminded myself to keep my back arched, and my tummy sucked in. I shook my ass a bit, swinging my hips back and forth in an exaggerated arc. Once I'd gotten used to the red lights and the volume of the music, I turned, putting my back against the mirror and arching again. You could work leaning against a wall or a mirror for entire songs, but I was curious about the pole and I wanted to show Desire I could connect with my customers. I'd learned about eye contact from Crystal, and it was true: Customers loved to feel *seen*.

I strutted downstage, ending up in front of the pole, standing over Joey. He drank his shot down in one gulp, holding it almost upside down over his mouth to get every single drop of whiskey. From the way he put his plastic shot glass down—regretfully, and with tender care—I guessed that he dearly wanted another. He wiped his mouth with the back of one big, rough hand and turned his full attention to me, his face carefully blank.

I put my back against the pole and slid down into a squat, giving him an eyeful of my panty-clad crotch. "Well," I said quietly. "This is awkward, isn't it?"

He laughed. The laughter shook the blank, set look out of his eyes. He blinked at me, and all of a sudden I knew he was actually observing me, instead of just keeping his face turned toward me but courteously absent, in order to satisfy Desire. "Howdy," I said.

"Well, hello, Lily," he said back, after cutting his eyes sideways to make sure Desire was only watching me dance, and not paying any attention to him. She stood behind the bar wiping glasses with a bar towel. She looked unimpressed, but then again, I hadn't done anything really interesting yet.

I kept moving, rolling forward from a squat into a kneeling position. I held up my boobs in Joey's face, presenting first one, then the other, then both together, creating cleavage.

I realized that I was feeling a strange sense of commonality with Joey. We were both working for Desire—I was trying to convince her to give me some shifts at Fancy's, and he was obediently impersonating a paying customer, to give my routine focus. But he wasn't licking his chops over my body, or appearing to feel any sense of power over me. We were both just drones—I was roboting away onstage, and he was sitting where he'd been told to sit.

Joey shook out a handkerchief and dragged it across his forehead.

"Getting too hot in here?" I asked.

"Huh? Yeah," he said, uncomfortably. I continued dancing in silence. Teasing him was mean—it was no fun to make him squirm.

The song was almost over and I hadn't taken my bra off, so I hung backward over the bar with my head nearly in Joey's lap, wrapping my thighs around the pole to keep myself from sliding off the stage, and reached behind my back to unhook myself. It was a tricky position, but the payoff would be that Desire's first view of my naked breasts would be them hanging upside down, looking as round and perky as fake tits. I released the clasp of my bra and tossed it toward the velvet curtain. I counted from ten down to one, then I used my stomach muscles to sit up. I glanced at Desire, cocking my head like *Do you want me to continue?*

"Nah, that's all right," she answered. "You're fine, babe. Go ahead and get dressed. We need day girls—can you work tomorrow, eleven to six?"

Yes, I could. I gathered my shed costume pieces, breathing hard from the exertion of the last part of my routine. I was in crappy shape—I'd grown lazy, sitting in the lounge of the Academy and ordering take-out with my friends. I'd gained weight—I could feel it around my midsection, and in my struggle to catch my breath after only one song. I hadn't danced in far too long. But a few weeks here and I'd be in fighting shape again, I knew.

"Yes, ma'am," I said. "You bet I can." I was grinning so hard my cheeks felt tight. A job! And I wasn't sure about Desire, but I thought I liked Joey. *A friend*—I tried that on. It felt a little strong. I was flustered at the idea of working with a *male* coworker, and trusting him as a friend. It seemed dangerous, like trying to domesticate a mountain lion.

Joey hadn't done anything customerish to me, nor was he in the strip club to purchase adult services—he was there to work. It would be grossly unfair of me to treat him like a customer. I wasn't about to put a collar on him and let him sleep by my bed, but I wasn't going to set out traps for him, either.

I went past the velvet curtain, down the rickety wooden steps, and into the dressing room, where I threw my pants and T-shirt on over my work thong and bra. I'd done it—I was really here, in New Orleans, and I had a job. I wanted to tell somebody, to have someone be proud of me, but there was nobody to tell who would understand. So I just crammed my high heels into my backpack and went out of the dressing room back into the club, to thank Desire for giving me a chance.

She and Joey sat at the bar, huddled in conversation. I noticed that she'd refilled his plastic shot glass. Desire held one of her own. A third plastic cup sat in front of an empty bar stool.

When Desire saw me coming out from under the green Exit sign, she called out, "Lily, hey Lily, come on over here, babe."

I hurried to the bar, grateful to be in my street shoes again. The carpet was a dangerous obstacle course. I knew it was only a matter of time before I tripped and went down onto my knees, or even worse. Knowing that I was going to trip wasn't like doing something about it—there was nothing to *be* done. Seven-inch heels plus bumpy carpet meant I was going to take a header and possibly end up flat on my back with cigarette butts in my hair. I hoped it wouldn't be on my first shift, when I'd be meeting some coworkers and trying to impress them with my big-city Pacific Northwest sophistication.

"Lily, here, have a shot, babe," croaked Desire, pushing the plastic shot glass of whiskey in my direction. "You earned it, girl. You got some nice little titties."

It wasn't even noon yet.

But what the hell, I figured. I was in New Orleans. And I'd just gotten a job. I lifted the glass and drank the shot in one motion, replacing the plastic cup on the bar crisply as the whiskey burned down my throat. I felt heat in my cheeks and willed myself not to cough.

Desire poured another generous shot into my cup. "There you go," she said.

It was useless to protest. Both she and Joey were looking at me with slightly glazed eyes and expectant smiles. It suddenly became clear to me that they were both sloshed. I'd only been in the dressing room for five minutes or so, but it didn't take long to drink shots of liquor from a bottle with a convenient pour-spout—especially not when your bartender poured with the heavy, practiced hand of the long-term alcoholic. My second shot sat in front of me, shimmering in the dusty gloom of the bar, topped by an oily film. It smelled like gasoline.

I hadn't eaten since the night before. I felt the first shot warming my belly, and almost immediately, my limbs began to feel warm and stretchy. I felt more comfortable in my clothes, too—all of a sudden the scratchy lace of my work bra was no longer irritating my skin, and the wet waistband of my pants seemed to expand and sit a little lower on my hips. I felt free and unconstricted. I seized the second shot, drank it before I could change my mind, and slammed my plastic cup back down on the bar again.

"So I was wondering, Lily, if you might start today instead of tomorrow," *Tah-marrah.* "Like, maybe, *now.*"

I was drunk enough that I didn't give her request a second thought. "Really? Yeah, I'd love to! I could really use the money."

Then I looked around. The club was dark. There were no customers, and no music was playing. Would there be any money to be made this early?

"Great! Because it's almost noon, and no other girls have shown up. I'll get in trouble with the owners if I run a shift with no girls," said Desire. "The dancers will probably start trickling in around three, but I need to have someone *now,* so I can open."

"Will there be customers?" I asked.

"Yeah," said Joey, speaking up for the first time since I'd come out to sit at the bar. "There will be. I just have to put on the sign and open the doors." He seemed relaxed and happy. I guessed he'd needed the shots Desire had poured him.

"Yeah, I'll do it," I said. "I'll go get dressed."

"Thank you, dolly," said Desire, smiling at me sweetly. The coral streak on her front teeth flashed like a warning. *Danger, danger!*

I giggled. I was loopy from the alcohol, and from the relief of finding work. Fancy's Foxhole had already come to feel familiar to me, and I could explore it more thoroughly once I'd gotten back into my work clothes.

Desire poured one more shot for herself, and one more for Joey. He looked at her pleadingly. "That one was small," he said. "Can you top it off?"

Desire clucked, but added a splash to Joey's shot. "That's all for now," she said. "We gotta work, babe."

He was already drinking. He gave no sign of having heard her, but he licked his lips and pushed back from the bar once his cup was empty.

I returned to the dressing room and got back into my slip, stockings, and high heels. I put on more powder, and more lip gloss. The whiskey had brought color to my cheeks. I really did look like the Little Dutch Boy, or a Campbell's Soup Kid. *M'm! M'm! Good!* I laughed.

Fluffing up my hair, I thought, *I am going to make so much money, so much money, so much money.* I repeated it like a mantra. Why was I going to make so much money? Because I was new, and because I was working the day shift, and because I was big and blond, and because I was just drunk enough to be able to conquer my natural shyness so I could talk to customers and get them to tip and buy dances.

I reminded myself to ask Desire if there were VIP shows here, and how much money to ask for them.

I hadn't brought anything to hold my money, but I figured I could stuff tips into the tops of my stockings and just transfer the money into my backpack frequently. I'd ask Desire if I could put my pack behind the bar. I didn't trust the lockers, and it would have been the height of stupidity to leave my things in an unattended dressing room open to girls I'd never met before. I had gotten spoiled at the Academy. I'd grown used to leaving my stuff around and having my friends keep it safe from would-be thieves—but that was there, in Seattle. I was known there. Nobody knew me here at Fancy's, and that made me prey until I made some alliances. I'd hide my stuff behind the bar until I made a few connections.

I spied a battered fashion magazine in one of the open lockers. I grabbed it and ripped out one of the pages. I used my black eyeliner pencil to write *55-C: Back in Black* on the glossy magazine paper, then went through the jukebox and jotted down a few other usable songs. Without the anxiety I'd felt before my audition interfering with my judgment, I was able to find a few more songs that I liked, or that I was at least familiar with. I could afford to be a little experimental now that I'd been hired—not as much rode on one song.

The songs on the jukebox at Fancy's were the exact opposite of what I was used to. They all seemed to be fast, frenetic, high-energy cuts, the kind of music you'd hear at a dance club or a rave. But I wasn't here to flashdance or shimmy up the pole like a monkey—I was here to stay low to the ground and sexy, and hopefully, to use my proximity to the customers to scoop up their money. I needed music that wouldn't interfere with my grifting.

"Hey there."

My head jerked up from the page. A black girl lounged in the doorway, observing me. Her head looked huge, but it was only because her weave was so full. She was dark-skinned and taller than me, with the broad shoulders, narrow hips, and long legs of a long-distance runner. She had a gym bag slung over one angular shoulder.

"Oh, hi," I said. I felt absurdly guilty, as if I'd been caught doing mischief. I hoped it hadn't been her magazine I'd ripped the page from. I didn't want to start off on the wrong foot and become known as someone who blithely damaged other workers' belongings.

"You new?" she said.

"Yeah," I said. We paused, trying to assess each other. I knew that it was best to stay terse—giving unnecessary information in an attempt to ingratiate myself would be viewed as weakness, and possibly exploited. I didn't know anyone here who would vouch for me, so I was in a dangerous position. If I gave the impression that I was soft, I'd be fucked with unmercifully. But if I acted too aggressive in my attempt to seem tough and powerful, the other girls would treat me as a dangerous threat. *Like going to jail,* I reminded myself. I kept my mouth shut, physically pressing my lips together to prevent myself from chattering or smiling.

"Where you from?" she asked.

"Seattle," I said.

I grabbed my backpack, making sure all my belongings were inside, and walked out of the dressing room without looking back.

"Devil's Plaything" — Danzig

I approached Desire, who was chopping garnishes at the bar. She looked up at me sharply.

"Who's the girl in the dressing room?" I asked casually.

"That's Kiara," she said. "She give you any problems?"

I was affronted. *"No,"* I said. Even if she had, I wouldn't have run to Desire to tattle. Did I look like I didn't know how to handle myself in a new dressing room? My chest expanded in indignation. I'd worked illegally, plying my trade in dumps that made Fancy's look like the Taj Mahal. I knew to keep my mouth shut for my first few days, until I could start making friends with the other girls and let down my guard a little. But even if nobody was friendly, you *never* went to management to resolve your conflicts with other girls.

Taking a deep breath, I suppressed my annoyance with Desire for treating me like a rank amateur. I felt the beginning of a headache from drinking so much whiskey on an empty stomach, and my stomach clenched with nausea.

"So, what's the stage fee?" I asked. The stage fee was what the house charged its dancers for the privilege of working. In Seattle, stage fees could be as high as $150 per shift. Dancers paid it because they had no other choice. Supposedly, they made enough money so that $150 wasn't a huge portion of their nightly income, but in reality, most clubs overhired in order to rake in dancer money, even when their business didn't justify the number of women they had on at any given time. You'd go into some venues and see twenty or thirty girls competing viciously for tip dollars from three or four customers.

The customers loved it because plenty of girls would perform illegal acts out of sheer desperation. Management loved it because it didn't matter how many customers came in during slow shifts—they were raking in most of their money from stage fees. It was unfair, but there was nothing to do but pay the money if you wanted to work.

"It's twenty a shift," said Desire. "It comes out of your drink money."

"Drink money?" *Oh, cool,* I thought. *B-drinking.* Fundamentally, B-drinking was getting customers to buy you high-priced "ladies'" drinks. I'd never done it before because in Seattle, alcohol wasn't allowed in adult entertainment venues. I knew B-drinking was illegal, but then again, so was touching dick for money.

"Single ladies' drinks cost nine, doubles are eighteen, and triples are twenty-seven," Desire told me. "The customer buys you a drink, says 'What you want, babe'—and you ask for as big a drink as you can get away with. You get two bucks a shot, so that's two for a single, four for a double, six for a triple. You gettin' this?"

I was.

"Do we have to drink them?" Three shots would put me on the floor. My stomach turned over sourly in protest at the very thought of drinking that heavily all night. The idea of getting tipsy with the customers seemed like a very, very bad idea.

Desire shrugged. "You drink 'em if you want to," she said. "If you don't drink 'em, they got no reason to buy you another."

Unfortunately, that made sense. I'd have to figure out a way to get around that. I knew I'd come up with something once I saw how the system worked—there was no way every girl working could drink that much, all night long. Somebody had to have a dodge that I could appropriate if I just kept my eyes open.

It seemed counterproductive to ask customers to buy us drinks instead of simply tipping us directly. The advantage to the bar was obvious. But then again, if the customer was uncomfortable tipping because he wanted to pretend that our interaction was primarily social instead of financial, the only way to pry money out of his wallet might very well be strong-arming him into buying a series of ladies' drinks. If our stage fees came out of our drink money, that was another very good reason to hustle drinks right there. Better that than the house insisting upon us paying cash at the beginning of every shift.

"What about private shows?" I asked. "Do you have a VIP?"

Desire pointed to the darkest corner of the bar, an area that seemed deliberately underlit and secluded. A row of chairs stood in a niche near the wall, and next to that was a small, enclosed area with solid wood planking up to waist level, topped with chicken wire. Squinting, I could see a sheet-covered couch in the little enclosure. Was there a little table, too? It was hard to tell.

"You see those chairs, babe?"

"Yeah."

"Okay, those are the regular VIPs. You take 'em over and do whatever you want—but keep your business to yourself. One song starts at thirty, and the house takes fifteen. But charge whatever you can get—either way, the house gets fifteen for one song, or thirty for three."

"What about the, uh . . ." I nodded toward the enclosure, which reminded me of a cross between the veal pens at Butterscotch's and the plastic boxes at Eros. Somebody had woven grimy plastic daisies through the chicken wire in an attempt to add perky charm to the enclosure—or, more probably, to decrease visibility. The fake flowers were a nice touch, I thought. If New Orleans Vice came around, the plastic daisies would just look like a pathetic attempt to add cheer to our work space, instead of a way to jerry-rig privacy for paid sexual interaction.

"That's the Special VIP. That's four hundred bucks for an hour, or two fifty for half an hour. Bar takes half."

I observed the couch with interest. The sheet covering it didn't look dirty, but then again, the towel-covered couches at Butterscotch's hadn't looked contaminated from a distance either. It was only once you got closer that you saw the couches were covered with dried, scaly patches of customer bodily waste. The customers didn't care—they stripped and wallowed in other men's semen happily. I didn't see a bottle of oil in the Special VIP pen, but that didn't mean one wasn't there. It was hard to see past the fake plastic flowers, I noticed approvingly.

"So, what's allowed in the Special VIPs?" For that kind of money I assumed we'd be flashing contraband views of what our G-strings covered, at the very least. I didn't expect Desire to spell that out, but I needed a sense of what management was willing to tolerate. I didn't want to come in as a new girl and immediately over- or underperform. Of course, anything Desire told me I'd take under advisement—I wouldn't know what other girls *really* did in there to make their money until I found an old girl I could trust.

Desire stared at me. She shrugged. "Just talk to them," she said. "Whatever. It's up to you. Or give 'em a little massage or somethin'. She looked at me blithely. "You know, like their shoulders."

I'd assumed I wouldn't be touching dick in New Orleans, but apparently it was still on the menu as an option. For half an hour at $250, with me making half, I'd get $125 for the same thing I was making $90 for at the Academy. And that had been for a full hour!

Of course, I could always just *talk to them*. One of the best-loved myths of the sex industry is that most customers just want conversation. In reality, they overwhelmingly prefer sexual mileage. They only talk when they believe that talking to their practitioner will result in extra service, when they're trying to make absolutely sure that they're receiving every minute of the time they're purchasing—or when they're Relaters trying to steal personal information so they can pretend to be friends, instead of customers.

"Oh yeah, and you gotta get 'em to tip the bar—a few bucks per song for VIP, and forty or fifty for the Special VIP. That way the bartender makes sure you aren't *disturbed*." Desire cocked a plucked eyebrow at me meaningfully.

I got it: a hush fee—money to look the other way. That was fine with me—I liked having all my business right out on the table like that.

I'm going to make so much money, so much money, my mind sang merrily. This was a lot of information to take in all at once, but I knew once I'd worked a few shifts it would all be second nature and I'd be able to hustle instinctively. There were so many ways to angle—the B-drinking, the VIPs, the tips to create covert, temporary alliances with the bar. I felt a hot rush of anticipation. Fancy's was like the Disneyland of the adult industry: Everywhere you looked, you saw another way to extract money from the customers. The club was one giant money-making machine—that is, if the clients didn't try to foil us by sitting at the stage rail and tipping stingily, dollar by dollar. Even so, a deadbeat could probably be pressured into buying at least a few drinks for a persistent girl.

"Tell him he gotta tip big in the Special VIP, and the bartender'll give him as many free drinks as he wants," Desire said.

"For real?"

"Yeah *for real*, Miss Seattle," said Desire, twisting her coral old-lady lips into a sly smile. "If they in there, they got money. We gotta treat 'em nice."

We looked at each other in sudden, cozy complicity. A drunk high roller was a man more interested in his dick than his wallet.

I was astonished at how much easier the availability of alcohol would make my job. I was also delighted by Desire's corrupt appreciation for the them-against-us nature of the industry.

Kiara emerged from the dressing room and flounced over to a side table, where she sat with her cell phone and proceeded to make call after call. She looked good—long, strong legs, a high ass, a nice six-pack stomach. She wore tiny white shorts, white go-go boots, and a little Dallas Cowboys cheerleader–style vest knotted under her breasts. If she'd been white, I would have been scared of her burying me financially. But the reality of the adult industry is that most customers prefer to spend their money on the kind of girls they see in porn and in mainstream rags like *Playboy,* which feature light-skinned black women only occasionally. Black adult performers have to be twice as polished and twice as ingratiating as their white counterparts, and even then, they make far less money for the same work. A dark-skinned woman like Kiara was at a huge disadvantage.

I envisioned a points system: I lost points for being chubby and tattooed, but gained points for being white and blond. I gained a few more points for my professional costume and stiletto-heeled shoes, though I lost a tick or two for having chin-length hair instead of a long mane. Kiara had points for her weave, her costume, and her toned body, but lost a bunch of them for being black, and a few more for being dark-complexioned. Some customers do prefer black women, but those men are few and far between. Even black customers often ignore black working girls and beeline for the girls with the most "points."

Blond hair or red hair are both strong positive points. The only ethnicity that gets more points than white is Asian, which is generally so point-heavy that if you're an Asian American worker, you can openly sport tattoos or have short hair and you'll still be a top earner. In some parts of the country, being Latina adds points; in other places it subtracts them. I figured it had to do with scarcity: In California and Texas, Latina girls are common, so that subtracts points. If those girls got smart and moved up to white, Nordic Minnesota to work, they'd rake it in as exotic senoritas.

If you're realistic about your points, you can vary your appearance to suit your own preferences without suffering a loss of income. For instance, I chose to take a hit on my points for my tattoos and my build, so I had to be stringent about maintaining my hair, makeup, and costumes. Some of your points you can control and others you can't—but working in the adult industry necessitates constant and brutal self-examination. You can't afford sentimentality: If you're at a points disadvantage, you either have to work your ass off to accrue points in other areas, or reconcile yourself to a reduced income.

I left Kiara alone and sat at another table by myself. Joey came out from the back weighted down with cases of beer, which he deposited on Desire's bar. Unlike me, he seemed energized by the whiskey he'd consumed. He whistled jauntily as he returned to the back for more beer, knocking on my table as he passed. "How you doing, Seattle?" he asked.

"All right," I said. In reality I was itchy and ill at ease. I needed to get started, to get my first customers out of the way, to make my first few dollars.

"All right, girls," called Desire from behind the bar. "Who's up first? I want to see your asses onstage."

Neither Kiara or I moved. There were no customers—what was the point? No working girl liked working for free. Dancing to an empty house would be silly, and a little bit humiliating.

"Kiara, babe, get your ass up there," said Desire. "Go every other song till we get some guys in here." She raised her voice. "Hey, Joey! Get on the door—*now!*"

He sped over to his post right outside Fancy's front door, under the cartoon fox ogling the phantom leg. "Hot girls," I heard him say to a group of tourists. It had to suck to stand outside in the New Orleans heat all day, trying to get other men to come in and spend money on adult entertainment. It was all the work of being a pimp with none of the status or income. No wonder he drank.

Kiara stood, stretching. Her costume looked like a bandage, covering her body in thin white strips. "44-G," she said loftily.

Desire punched the numbers into a battered black metal box mounted behind the bar on the wall.

Kiara had picked a rap song. I had no idea of the artist and couldn't make out any of the words except for *Bring 'em out, bring 'em out, bring 'em out,* repeated over and over on top of a heavy beat, with synthesizers *bleep*ing and *bloop*ing in the background.

I was curious to see Kiara's routine, so I moved to a table near the Special VIP enclosure where I could see the stage and the front door. If anyone walked in, I'd know. The plastic daisies looked funereal in the dim haze of the club, floating like ghosts in the dark.

Kiara was on the pole near the ceiling, hanging upside down like a bat. As I watched, she loosened her thighs and slid down to the floor of the stage, supporting her weight on her palms. From there she cartwheeled off the pole, ending in a standing position like an Olympic gymnast in a medal-winning dismount. She wasn't even breathing hard as she seized the pole again, leaping against it and spinning as she ascended to the ceiling, as if gravity were something she had simply chosen to disregard.

By the end of her song I was entranced. Kiara was an athlete, and watching her was a privilege. I dreaded watching customers tuck dollars into her costume. How could they ever pay her enough for her abilities? She needed lucrative corporate sponsorship and a Wheaties contract, not a few limp dollar bills. I wasn't looking forward to going up after Kiara. I wasn't a bad dancer, but my lackluster booty-shaking was no match for her strength, daring, and grace.

The front door opened, letting in a bright slash of sunlight and a sudden burst of noise from Bourbon Street. Two middle-aged white men with identical bulging guts staggered in, clutching beverages in plastic hand-grenade-shaped containers. The drinks appeared to be bright green and were consumed through long plastic straws that bristled out of the bellies of the grenades. The men were riotously drunk. They peered owlishly into the gloom of the bar, rocking on their feet and howling with laughter. Desire straightened behind the bar, throwing out her chest.

"What'll you-all have today, gentlemen?" she asked. "We gotta one-drink minimum to watch the show." She nodded toward Kiara, who was pretzeling herself into a complicated, crablike position midway up the pole, imperiously giving no sign of having noticed the men at the door.

"Aw, shit, brown sugar," complained one man loudly. His words were so slurred it sounded like his tongue had been stung by a hornet, or shot full of novocaine. If I hadn't known he was drunk, I would have assumed he was retarded.

"You all got any white girls working?" his friend asked Desire in a heavy Southern accent. Overcome, the two men guffawed, poking and slapping each other in their respective guts. Bright green liquid sloshed onto the carpet. Their smell reached me all the way across the room. They smelled pickled, marinated in alcohol like fetal pigs—as if they'd been drinking nonstop for days. I drew back into the shadows—I wanted to watch them a bit before I approached. Besides, my eyes were watering and my head was throbbing in a dull, thuddy pulse. I breathed shallowly, trying not to taste their lighter fluidy fumes. I imagined lighting a match and incinerating them both.

"Yeah, we got a hot blond girl, name of Lily," said Desire. "She's up next. What can I get you? Shots?"

"Shit," said the first man, climbing onto a stage bar stool labor-iously. "I'll have—what the fuck will I have?" He addressed his friend in consternation. "I got a Grenade already, Earl!" Suddenly he belched—a long, fruity *brrrrrrrrrap*. The two men roared.

"You'll have—we'll have—two Millers," said Earl. "You got it ice-cold?"

"Yeah," said Desire. It was as if a curtain had been pulled across her face. Her expression was unreadable, betraying no opinion.

The first man—I had come to understand he was the drunker of the two—sat watching Kiara impassively, swaying from the waist up. She dropped off the pole lightly—*like a spider,* I thought—and approached him, smiling and holding her shorts away from her body for a tip. He ignored her. "Hey, where's my drink?" he yelled to his buddy, who stood at the bar, entranced by Desire's bosom.

Kiara's song ended and she stood there for a moment, waiting for her tip. A customer who sat at the stage was expected to give at least a few dollars to every entertainer out of courtesy, to pay for his coveted position of proximity. A customer who sat at the stage and didn't tip was sending a clear message of disrespect. Eventually, after a long, awkward pause, Kiara turned on her heel and walked offstage without glancing back.

I was up. I stood clumsily, pushing away from the table and staggering as my heel caught on the carpet.

"Lily, do two," called Desire.

The two customers echoed her in jaunty fellowship, cackling.

"Yeah, Lily, do two!" said Earl. He seized the two Millers he'd paid for and brought them over to his friend, placing them on the counter with deliberate, drunken care.

"You can do *us* two," responded his seated friend. They brayed laughter, clinking their beer bottles together to celebrate their own irresistible wit. Then they settled in, huddling together in bleary anticipation. Plastic Grenade cups sat, forgotten, at their feet.

Joey appeared from outside. He approached Desire, cocking his head at the two drunks waiting by the stage. She shook her head. Joey shrugged. He took a moment to cool off under the air-conditioning, mopping his forehead with his handkerchief, then went back to his post. "Hot girls," I heard him say again. *Yeah, hot girls and two disgusting, smelly drunks,* I thought.

When I emerged from behind the velvet curtain, I called my selections out to Desire and then immediately approached the two men, dropping to my knees in front of them. "How you-all doing today?" I asked sweetly, in my brand-new Southern accent. "You boys havin' a real good time?"

They grunted, nodding.

"Now, don't tell me you're shy," I said. "Big ol' men like you; don't tell me you're scared of a little girl like me." I giggled.

If I didn't get them on my side right away, I knew they'd sit and talk about me as if I weren't there. They had to know I could hear them, and that I could see them the same way they could see me. I had to be different than a porn DVD. I had to get them to engage—not as overgrown schoolboys who could sit back sniggering and making loutish cracks about me, but as men who felt a proprietary sense of protectiveness over my body. Ultimately my goal was to make them feel more powerful than me. Most men loved being chivalrous to women who were meekly grateful to them for their patronage. But if I seemed *too* weak, they'd feel sorry for me, and while I'd avoid harassment, I also wouldn't be making the kind of tips a more assertive girl could command. The ideal combination was like sweet-and-sour sauce: I had to be both spunky *and* vulnerable.

"Why, I'm more nervous than you-all are!" I cooed. "After all, this is *my* first time in a strip club—but I bet you gentlemen have been around the block once or twice."

They laughed, punching each other in the shoulders and chest.

"We want to see some titties!" said the drunker of the two. He slammed his beer bottle down and howled.

"I don't know if I've got any of those today, gentlemen," I said primly. "I can check our stockroom."

Earl guffawed in delighted surprise. His eyes lifted to my face for a moment, then slid back to my chest. I'd made contact.

"You hush up," he said to his friend. "You let Miss Lily do her thing." He nodded at me. "You go on now, girl."

"Why thank you, gorgeous," I said. I reached out and briefly cupped Earl's face with my palm, holding my breath so as not to accidentally inhale any air that had spent any time inside either of them. "All right, now this is my first day, so you-all be kind, now." I stood and stepped back to the mirror, leaning against it and arching my back.

After a little while, both Earl and his friend retrieved their wallets and began laying out singles methodically, as if hypnotized. They didn't speak to each other. It was as if the foreplay of their fun and games was over, and now they were there to buckle down to the serious study of my body. I arched, flexed, bent, and strutted as best I could. I really didn't have to do much. When I was tired, I just struck a pose and held it, either clinging to the pole or leaning against it. I did a lot of deep squatting, hanging from the pole with one hand and leaning back. It felt good to stretch my back like that, and while I was in that position, I could think about what I wanted to do next. By the end of my second song I was simply lying on my side on the stage floor, topless, plucking dollars from the two drunks' fingers and giggling. They didn't seem to notice any qualitative difference between my performance and Kiara's.

By the time I was done I'd made handfuls of dollars—mostly ones, but a few fives were stuck in there as well.

I passed Kiara on the wooden stairs as she went up to do her set, and we both looked away. I refused to insult her by attempting to offer her any commiseration, but I felt horrible about her having to go out and perform for those two rednecks. We weren't friends, though. Any kind words on my part would necessarily be suspect.

As I reentered the showroom, I saw Kiara up at the top of the pole like a treed kitten, avoiding the two slavering hound dogs beneath.

"Layla"—
Derek and the Dominos

Fancy's was the most traditional place I'd ever worked. When you said *stripper* or *adult entertainer,* most people envisioned a place more or less like Fancy's, not like the Academy or even Butterscotch's. Fancy's had a stage, a pole, and a bar. Women danced, made tips, and tried to sell private shows. Working there was like being a stripper in a movie. And I wasn't just *any* stripper—I was a stripper on Bourbon Street, America's world-famous red-light district. I felt like part of an elite group of super strippers, like we should be wearing capes and fighting for justice.

I was onstage one afternoon about six weeks after my hire, going through my paces. A few clumps of men sat around the stage and I rotated through them, approaching each group of buddies and giving them a different pose. A group of black men at one end of the bar liked ass and doggy-style stuff, but they weren't tipping very well so I breezed right past them after a perfunctory shimmy.

"Hey girl, come back here. Shit! What's the matter, you don't like brothers?"

"I like brothers who tip, baby," I called back sweetly. I didn't necessarily want to drive them off—I planned on coming out after my set to see if I could get any of them to buy a private show—but my hopes weren't high. They were locals, not tourists. Tourists came to Fancy's with lots of money to spend and no idea of what local adult services cost, and best of all, they were generally crocked on the cheap daiquiris being sold up and down the street from storefronts and makeshift lean-tos. Locals, on the other hand, usually came to bars like Fancy's to nurse inexpensive drinks and greedily eyeball as many tits and asses as they could without tipping.

Despite my chiding, none of the brothers proffered a tip, so I shrugged and continued moving away from them. I heard a chorus of groans behind me.

"Shit, she *racist*," I heard.

I turned back. "Hey, fuck you, man," I said lightly. "I'm not racist. You just don't know how to treat a lady." I smiled and slapped my own ass, letting it jiggle temptingly. You never knew—they might have a few extra dollars for me on my next stage rotation. I wasn't too proud to be grateful for two or three crumpled dollar bills.

Local *or* tourist, black customers tended to love me, with my big white ass and my überblond helmet of porn star hair. But I wasn't working because I needed to feel admired. I couldn't afford to humor customers who weren't tipping, even the local working-class heroes with whom I ordinarily felt professional kinship. My rent was coming up. I had come in needing to make $250, and so far I'd only made $19 from stage tips. I couldn't afford any bad investments of time or energy in customers who weren't actively increasing my income.

I put my hands on the mirror and arched my back, eliciting predictable howls from the knot of nontippers at the end of the bar. That was enough ass stuff for them—I had already been too generous. I turned and put my back against the mirror, surveying the other customers and trying to guess which ones might be game for a private show. I hated being touched, but I needed the money badly. I set my sights on the lone white man sitting at the end of the bar, opposite the boisterous locals.

I approached and knelt on the wooden stage floor directly in front of him. Spreading my knees apart, I leaned back as far as I could, firmly placing one hand on my inner thigh, directly adjacent to my crotch. I could hear the cartilage in my knees pop as I rested for a moment, deliberately stretching my back and breathing deeply in a kind of stripper yoga I liked to do when I didn't have a large number of customers to entertain and could afford to move slowly. Once I'd settled into my new pose, I began pumping my hips up and down in a languid fucking motion. The customer in front of me stared at my crotch avidly, laying dollar bills under my ass, one by one. The bills stuck to my ass cheeks, but I didn't break my pose to peel them off.

"Oh, thank you, baby," I purred, stroking my thigh as if my clit were located just above the lacy edge of my stocking. *No messing around in your panties,* Desire had said, and I respected that. Fake masturbation was a surefire tip generator at Fancy's—I just made sure to locate my activity slightly off-center so as to obey the letter of the law, if not the spirit.

I tried moaning softly. The customer in front of me reddened, then placed a five-dollar bill on top of the pile of ones underneath me.

"You like that, baby?" I said. I clambered into another position, using my pose change as an opportunity to peel a damp bill from my bare ass. I added it to the pile. I looked forward to spending it. *Here, have some stripper ass-sweat with that dollar!* The more I worked in the sex industry, the more I believed that people who held money between their teeth for any reason were lunatics.

I decided on doggy style with my knees far apart, in order to display the strip of fabric covering my crotch and asshole to best advantage. If my customer liked pussy shows, I'd give him the pussy show of his dreams. I sank into my pose, pressing my chest to the floor in a strippery Downward Dog. My back popped like Rice Krispies.

I heard groaning from the other end of the stage.

"Aw, *shit!* Bring that ass back over here, girl!"

I ignored them. My money was clearly on the lone white man. Couldn't they see the pile of ones and fives between my seven-inch platform heels?

I was a little surprised to realize that I was no better or worse a stage dancer than any of the other girls at Fancy's. Stage dancing wasn't like real dancing, though—it was more like slowed-down vogueing, a series of poses ideally, but not necessarily, oiled with graceful transitions. It was a lot like posing for porn—find a position, and hold. Find another position, and hold. And another, and hold. You had to give the customers a chance to see you, and to appreciate the pornographic potential of each pose. If you moved too fast, they missed all the good stuff and were merely left with a hazy impression of whirling movement. Most clients were accustomed to porn, used to pausing their adult entertainment at will for closer examination. You had to work with their expectations.

I braced my knees and clenched the big muscles of my thighs, making my ass and legs shake tantalizingly. I'd stolen that move from another dancer at Fancy's—it felt gross, but men seemed to love seeing girl-flesh tremble. I thought I could understand that— it was a biological imperative for heterosexual men to be attracted to women who looked reproductively viable, and nothing looked healthier or more sexually fit than a well-nourished woman with enough flesh to jiggle. I was continually amazed by women who dieted in order to become as gaunt as fashion models in hope of attracting mates. The only thing diets did was inspire more men to go to strip clubs.

My song ended, and I struggled to my feet. Getting up from a floor position in platform heels was difficult, and looking good doing it was almost impossible. A few more fives were on top of my little snowdrift of money, and I tucked them into the lace band of my stocking carefully.

"Shall I come out and join you?" I asked my pussy-show customer. He shrugged, suddenly shy now that no music was playing.

"I'll take that as a yes, cowboy," I said. I thought of my rent, and treated him to a dazzling grin. *I am sexy,* I thought. *You want me.* I tried to give the impression that I'd be up for illegal touch, for not very much money.

I guided him back toward the bar, where I slid Desire a five-dollar bill. "Here you go, gorgeous." *Help me, please,* I said to her with my eyes, deliberately shifting my gaze to the customer by my side.

"Hiya, Lily," she said flirtatiously. "You looked so hot up there. Din't she look hot, babe?"

My customer hemmed and hawed. "Yeah," he said finally.

"You wanna buy the lady a drink? Lily, what you want, babe?"

"I'd love a drink. I'll have my usual double Absolut. Is that all right, darling?" I pressed my breasts against my customer's arm, looking up into his face. I made sure to keep my lips wet and parted—a cocksucker's mouth, glossed with frosty pink.

Cum lips, Viva had called it. Customers loved cum lips. I assumed this love was another aspect of their apparent fascination with other men's semen.

I licked my cum lips eagerly and smiled. "A double's okay? I'm really thirsty." *Thirsty for cum,* I thought. It was psychic warfare. I was convinced that if I thought things loudly enough, the customers would pick up on my astral vibrations and respond without being conscious of any manipulation on my part, the way subliminal advertising sold liquor with pictures of naked women's bodies in the ice cubes.

My customer nodded helplessly, pulling two twenties out of his wallet. I peered into it as best I could. It looked pretty full, though it was hard to discern denominations. I noted that he put it into the front pocket of his jacket, instead of his back hip pocket. *Good boy.* I smiled. If I could nab a private show, I'd be sure to slip my hands in and—

Oh my god, I thought suddenly. *I'm a career criminal.*

I paused for a moment, considering. I hadn't been raised to pick pockets, like some kind of Dickensian waif—but then again, I wasn't even supposed to be here in New Orleans, at Fancy's or at any other adult establishment. And yet, here I was.

If I got caught jacking a customer's wallet, I'd be fired.

But Desire didn't even know my real name, and Bourbon Street was full of other strip clubs. I'd do all right. Besides, I wouldn't *be* caught.

Fuck it—I had to pay my rent.

"That's eighteen for the ladies' drink, and five for the beer." Desire busied herself making change.

I grinned, and clinked my plastic shot glass against my customer's beer bottle. "Shall we go sit down?" I asked. He followed me meekly. *You're trapped, pussy boy,* I thought.

I picked a table against the back wall, in a niche near the VIP area. The light was dimmest back there, and I could see the stage from where I sat. I picked the seat closest to the wall so Desire couldn't see me from behind the bar. It was all about visibility at Fancy's—who could see you, who couldn't, who you could see, and what you did with that information. Like cats, we constantly maneuvered for sheltered vantage points from which to observe the action on the floor.

My customer drank from his bottle as I sipped from my plastic cup delicately, as though it were filled with Absolut rather than the plain water I'd had Desire put in my cup.

"What's your name, darling?" I asked.

"Cooper," he said. He drank again.

"You here on vacation, honey?" I spoke slowly in my syrupy Southern accent. Some days it crept over into a quasi-Midwestern twang, which sounded even more earnest and dim-witted. Women despised dumb men, but men seemed to find mild mental retardation as arousing as fancy lingerie. You really couldn't go wrong wearing a push-up bra while giving the impression of clinical idiocy—it was the classic one-two punch, demonstrated with great efficacy by women like Anna Nicole Smith and Marilyn Monroe.

"Yeah," said Cooper. He began shredding his cocktail napkin into strips.

I guessed he was about forty—paunchy, with thinning hair and the doughy body of a man who sits at a desk to earn his money.

Cooper stared down at his pile of napkin strips. I was suddenly tempted to suggest weaving a paper pot holder to bring home as a souvenir for his wife—it would be a little piece of Fancy's Foxhole she could enjoy every time she took a pan of fish sticks out of the oven.

"You want to drink up?" I lifted my plastic shot glass naughtily. If we pounded our drinks, he would have to buy us another round.

Cooper shrugged, then abruptly seized his beer bottle and upended it. I tossed my "shot" to the back of my throat neatly, and swallowed.

"*Oh,*" I said, crinkling my nose. "It burns."

You had to be smart about B-drinking—attention to detail was what made it work. If the customers suspected you weren't drinking alcohol or weren't getting drunk enough, they'd stop buying ladies' drinks—but if you were careful to act progressively more inebriated with every drink, they'd buy them all night in the hope of getting you messed up enough to fuck them, or at least give them a drunken, dirty VIP. Few customers could resist the temptation of getting extra service from a stripper too impaired to enforce her usual professional boundaries.

"Can I have another, baby?" I asked, standing and playfully flipping my skirt up to favor Cooper with a brief flash of satin panty, since he'd seemed so captivated by them before. Cooper reached out, as if mesmerized, and tried to touch my panty-clad crotch. I skillfully turned my hip, deflecting his hand.

"I'll go and fetch you another beer. Here—give me a little money, sugar. No reason for you to wait in line." I giggled, hoping he wouldn't point out that there was no line at the bar. Desire stood alone, leaning against the counter and wiping out a glass with a bar rag.

He reached into his jacket and extracted two more twenties. That was good to know—all twenties. My guess was that he'd hit an ATM before coming to Fancy's. I was suddenly energized, on point. *Don't fuck this up,* I told myself.

I frisked off to the bar, my stupid plaid skirt so short that I felt cool air on my ass.

"Desire, two more, please," I said.

"He gonna get a private show with you?" asked Desire, twisting the cap off Cooper's beer and plunking it down onto a paper bar napkin next to my ersatz double Absolut.

"Yeah, I'm pretty sure," I said. "I gotta seal the deal. He's shy."

I paid her, tipping her $5 of Cooper's money. I tucked the rest of the money into my stocking. If Cooper asked for his change I could always pull it out again, pretending I'd put it there for safekeeping.

I remembered something I'd seen other girls do. "Can I have a little vodka in the bottom of a shot cup, Desire?" I asked. When she passed the cup across the bar, I dipped my fingers in it and anointed my hair, neck, and cleavage with liquor as if I were crossing myself with holy water. That would ensure that I returned to Cooper smelling like a distillery. I finished by sprinkling a few drops on my tongue—wincing as the raw alcohol incinerated my taste buds—to make sure that my breath carried the scent of liquor as well. I'd ride the St. Charles streetcar home from the French Quarter tonight smelling like a late-stage alcoholic, but in the hard-drinking city of New Orleans, I would be merely one of many.

I needed to get back to Cooper to strong-arm him into a private show before some other girl sidled up to him and stole the session that I'd earned by laying all the groundwork. He was at a crucial, unprotected point: drunk, but not too drunk, and horny, thinking about panties or crotches or whatever it was he liked when he stared between a dancer's legs. It was up to me to sell him an expensive show. If I didn't do it just right, though, he could feel pressured—and a pressured customer would bolt. I had to be light and flirtatious, as if the money were merely an awkward formality between him and management. I needed to give the impression that I was so into him I'd do a VIP for free if they didn't make me charge. He'd bought me two ladies' drinks, and I appreciated that—but now it was time to go in for the kill.

"Hey Desire, actually, can I have a shot?" I asked. I needed to relax so I could strike the right playful, sexy chord with Cooper. Alcohol would help. "Jack's, up?"

She shrugged and poured a double shot of bourbon into another plastic shot glass. Desire never charged me for liquor, probably because I paid her to substitute water or soda for the alcohol in my drinks most of the time. When I *did* want to drink she poured heavily—and even so, the bar still ended up way ahead. I wondered how the owners accounted for Fancy's sky-high liquor sales when they weren't spending an appropriate amount of money to replace their stock. Or maybe all strip clubs cooked their books—it would be tempting, considering how large a percentage of their profits was in cash.

I tossed my shot back and felt warmth spreading across my chest almost instantaneously. Drinking made working at Fancy's much easier. I was a better dancer with a few shots of liquor in me, and I was able to be more gracious to the customers. When I sold private shows, liquor allowed me to detach and let my mind roam free, instead of being grounded in the loathing I felt as my customers pawed my breasts and ass.

I'd also discovered that drinking with the customers was not as abhorrent as I'd thought it would be—as long as I didn't get falling-down drunk, I could have a shot or two and not impair my own money-making ability. In fact, I seemed to do better when I was tipsy. Liquor quieted my brain and allowed me to work on autopilot—it was like a big, fluffy, soothing blanket that wrapped around me and kept me warm and loose, muffling my tendency toward constant analysis.

I thanked Desire, picked up Cooper's bottle of beer and my tap water, and made my way back to our table.

"99 Problems" — Jay-Z

I placed Cooper's beer in front of him and took my seat against the wall, smoothing my skirt down behind me to create a layer of protection between my bare ass and the stained, fabric-covered seat. It was unpleasant to think about how many other working girls had occupied that chair before me. Was I sitting on layered stripes of pasty white vaginal secretions, pubic nits, crab eggs, streaks of shit? Was it possible to contract herpes from a chair?

I'd been going in for full-spectrum STD testing every six months since I first started working at Butterscotch's, paying extra to be tested for both kinds of herpes and getting my cervix swabbed for evidence of human papilloma virus. I'd never contracted anything, but that didn't ease my mind. I was still phobic about other people's bodily juices.

I sipped my water daintily. "Oh my gosh, I have to slow down. I don't want to get *too* drunk, and I'm already buzzed."

"You are?" Cooper stared down at his beer bottle. "Well, have another." I felt heat and pressure on my thigh. I looked down. He'd put his hand on my leg! *Why Cooper, you old rogue.* His beers must have kicked in. I pressed my knees together so he couldn't go kamikaze and slide his hand up to my pussy.

I giggled, putting my hand over my mouth. "I think I have a better idea. Do you see those chairs over there, against the wall?"

"Yeah," he said. He still wouldn't look at me, but he prodded my thigh as if checking it for ripeness. *If you run my stockings I will punch you, Cooper.*

"Well, you wanna go over there and mess around?" I whispered. "It's fun, and it's only forty dollars for one song, plus a tip to the bartender so she'll make sure we have privacy." I held my breath. I'd started high—if he demurred, I'd knock my price back to the house standard, $30. "You can tip me, too, baby— I love getting really naughty."

"I don't know," he said.

The whiskey made me brave. "Oh, come on," I cajoled. "You gotta get a lap dance to tell the guys about at home, right?" I sighed. "And I'm *so horny.*"

Cooper sat in silence, a leaden, man-size lump of need and hesitation. He wanted it—I knew he did—but he was waiting for a hard sell, so he could avoid taking responsibility for his own lust.

I was sick of playing around—if Cooper needed to feel forced, I had to be more aggressive. I reached under the table and brushed his crotch with my hand. I couldn't tell if he was hard or not.

I gambled. "Ooh," I said. "Is that big thing for me?"

"Yeah," he said. Suddenly he shoved his hand into his breast pocket and seized his wallet. "Let me get one song," he said, extracting two twenty dollar bills. I tucked the money into my stocking top. "How much do you want to give the bartender, sugar? I'll go bring it to her."

Cooper fished around in his pants and pulled out a wad of ones. He peeled off four with a flourish, and handed them to me. He drained his beer and replaced the empty bottle on the table, belching.

"Okay, honey, meet me over there," I said, pointing to the VIP area. "Pick your favorite chair, and I'll be right back." He looked doubtful. "I'm just going over to the bar to square everything up with the house, honey—I promise I'll be right back." Now that he'd committed, he seemed to be suffering from separation anxiety. Or maybe he was afraid of me running right out the front door with his precious $40—like I'd get far on my crippling platform shoes! I couldn't even walk on the carpet in Fancy's, let alone make time on the cobblestones outside!

I imagined myself with a broken ankle, being shot like a wounded horse. The thought wasn't as funny as I'd hoped it would be. What *did* happen to us, when our bodies gave out? What would happen to me? Suddenly I felt a savage stab of need. I needed money. I needed as much money as I could get, because money was the only thing that would allow me to grow old with some dignity.

Strippers aren't greedy, I thought. *We're just scared.*

I reached the bar and counted out fifteen dollars plus Desire's four-dollar tip. "You want another shot?" she asked. I hesitated.

"Why not?" I said. I gulped the Jack Daniels down. Four shots in five minutes and I couldn't even feel them. *My tolerance must be getting really out of control,* I thought. But I needed it to do a private show. I couldn't do it sober—I'd tried, and it was nearly impossible. Alcohol was the palliative I needed—a warm fuzzy blanket to muffle my feelings, so I could relax and act sexy. Plus I really needed to quit thinking about being shot.

Let it go, I thought. *Just let it go. Laisser le bon temps* fucking *rouler.* Let the good times roll.

I had a job to do.

I lurched back to the VIP area, unsteady as usual on my heels. Cooper had chosen a seat in the middle of the row and lounged there awkwardly, his arms frozen across the tops of the neighboring chairs in a transparent attempt to look casual and relaxed. I climbed onto Cooper's lap, straddling him heavily to keep him fixed in place, and placed his hands around my waist. Pulling his face to my chest, I noticed he had little white flakes of dandruff glued to his oily scalp and scattered throughout his mouse-colored hair.

I used my hands to push my boobs together. Cooper moaned and pushed his face against them, burrowing into my chest like an infant. I heard the beginning of Kiara's song, the one about bringing them out. Was that a long song? I couldn't remember.

Cooper was muttering something into my skin.

"What, baby?" I asked, pulling my chest back a few inches.

"I want to make you feel good," he said. He slid his hands from my waist to my bottom, lifting my skirt and cupping my ass cheeks in his hands. His fingers scrabbled at my G-string.

Ugh. I could feel his erection through his pants. It felt like a tiny animal, rearing its little head and demanding attention. Muzzling my disgust, I kept my weight on it.

"You're making me feel good already," I responded by rote.

You know what would really make me feel good, Cooper? Sawing your cock off with a rusty tin can lid. But my violent ideation was habitual, not personal. I bore Cooper no particularly vicious ill will. He was just a customer, like any other. They were interchangeable and equally loathsome.

I thought of Joey sitting at the stage for my audition, uncomfortably slumped over his liquor, hating having to impersonate the kind of man who would sit at a stage and watch a stranger disrobe for dollars. He'd never once made me feel anything other than fully human, though he'd seen me nearly naked and pretending to finger my pussy onstage. Why did some men become customers, while others didn't? Why were some men born with the innate ability to treat other people as interchangeable masturbation devices, while others weren't?

Stalling, I slowly untied my shirt, tossing it onto the chair next to us. When I couldn't waste any more time, I reached behind myself and unhooked my bra, grimly placing it on top of my shirt. Delighted, Cooper began licking my chest. He licked down to my nipple, paused, then licked that too. I could smell his spit, warm and yeasty from beer. I felt a predictable wave of nausea in my belly, strong and hard.

I hated having my breasts sucked, but all the other girls at Fancy's allowed that in their VIPs and my own sick loathing didn't seem like a good enough reason to buck the trend. It was *all* disgusting. If I didn't let them mess with my boobs, it was a short, steep slope to not letting them touch me at all, and from there I'd tumble into wanting to strangle them for even looking at me—and that would put me out of work. I usually did my best to entertain with words instead of mileage, but VIP shows were all about touch, not my usual smoke and mirrors. As Cooper nursed from my teat I simply checked out, hanging an imaginary For Rent sign in the vacant space behind my eyes, trying to disconnect the nerves in my skin so I only felt his invasion as pressure, nothing more than that. I went limp and concentrated on breathing in, counting to five, then breathing out, counting to five, while Cooper licked and pawed my body until the song was over.

At the end of the song, Cooper bought three more songs for $100.

The disgust and rage I experienced during Cooper's endless four songs overloaded my circuits until they simply failed, blowing me out like a light bulb or a radio transistor. I'd pushed through countless layers of humiliation and sadness and anger and found, to my relief, that what was on the other side was simply absence of feeling. I realized I could fuck or suck or lick balls like Princess Lavender, and it would all mean pretty much the same thing, which was nothing.

Also, I was plastered. I went up for my next stage set and spent both songs walking up and down the bar, picking my way past drinks and ashtrays, pausing every now and again to squat down and let a customer tuck a tip in the side of my G-string. The customers didn't seem to notice I wasn't dancing or even attempting to pose.

Later that shift, I sold a half-hour Special VIP show to a customer who tipped Desire $50 to bring us a tray of Jägermeister shots. I sat on the couch in the Special VIP pen and let him jerk off to me. He was having a difficult time achieving orgasm because he was so drunk, so I distracted him by offering him more alcohol from Desire's bar tray.

"You drink some," he slurred. "I want *you* to have a nice time, too."

I thought of all the ways I could be having a nice time. None of them included sitting on a sheet-covered couch behind a wall of dusty plastic daisies, drinking with a customer.

"Okay," I said. I lifted the plastic shot glass to my lips but kept them tight, and then as soon as his gaze slid away from me I dumped the Jäger onto the floor, using my shoe to rub it into the carpet. It left a dark stain, but nobody would notice.

While my customer downed more Jägermeister, I straddled him, avoiding the limp, dead worm of his cock, and ran my hands over his chest. I felt the bulge of his wallet in his breast pocket, and savagely pinched his nipple.

"Ow," he said thickly.

"Oh, sorry, baby," I said, rubbing his chest with the flat of one hand while blatantly extracting his wallet with the other. I dropped it on the floor in one smooth motion, and used the platform of my shoe to kick it under the couch. I felt unstoppable, like a super criminal coolly moving on instinct alone—as if I could freeze time or make things occur through the sheer force of my own will. I slipped my nipple into my customer's mouth to reward him for not noticing the missing weight of his wallet. He sucked gratefully, his mouth as sticky and stained as the carpet beneath my feet.

It occurred to me that my Special VIP customer was making out with Cooper via my chest. We were all squishing up and into and against each other, like amoebas; we were all trapped in a rich slurry of spit and cum and vaginal slime, and we were all culling and greedily devouring each other's waste. I was a greasy bone being passed back and forth between gleeful dogs, their muzzles slobbery with the taste of each other's assholes. I was only involved as a kind of human serving platter, and that was what the men who came to places like this wanted women like me to be, because it excited them to have access to each other and because, I suspected, they enjoyed the idea that some women could be paid to facilitate that access.

My Special VIP customer moaned and shuddered as he chafed his penis with his hand, jerking it roughly from the root of his pubic hair. He took his mouth off my breast for a moment, spat into his own palm for lubrication, and latched back on to my nipple. I waited for him to finish.

I gazed past the plastic daisies with some difficulty, observing Kiara on the regular VIP chairs with a customer. She squirmed on his lap and then suddenly his tongue was in her mouth and they were kissing. Kissing! Despite my numbness, I felt a brief flutter of contempt and revulsion. But then again, I didn't have the moral high ground. We were all rolling in shit, working it between our fingers and rubbing it into our hair. The shit Kiara was gulping down was no worse than the shit my customer was smearing all over my chest, which was no worse than the shit he'd squeeze out into his own palm when he came.

I looked away. I thought of the word *unclean.* This place was unclean. I guessed that when women did this kind of work and didn't take care of one another, we ended up struggling through filthy, stinking rivers of customer shit by ourselves, desperately trying to keep ourselves afloat. Maybe sometimes it was easiest just to let ourselves go under.

My Special VIP customer finally shot his load into his own hands. He wanted to keep lapping saliva off my chest, but I convinced him to have more Jägermeister instead. While he drank I called Joey over and asked him to put my client into a cab, because he'd been a little bit overserved—even by New Orleans standards—and needed to sleep off his intoxication. My Special VIP didn't protest. He was tired, close to passing out, and his hands were covered in the pearly stew of his own ejaculate. Joey looked at my customer's hands and then at me, and I thought he looked sad. But I was so distant that he just looked small and far away, like a sad person on TV.

I scurried back to the Special VIP pen and felt under the couch for the wallet. Once I'd retrieved it, I shoved it down the front of my panties, under my skirt, and beelined for the women's bathroom, where I locked myself into a stall for privacy. My heart was pounding. It was like Christmas, and the wallet was a present I was about to unwrap. I felt no sense of moral conflict over my theft. The customers weren't really people to me—they were just sets of grasping hands, hungry mouths, and insistent pricks. I had no illusions about any sense of commonality or honor between working girls and our customers—they were there to get what they could out of us, and we were there to get what we could out of them. Just because I'd won this round didn't mean I wouldn't be tricked or hurt by a customer the next time I worked. I hadn't started the war, but I'd fought well in this particular battle, and I deserved the spoils.

His wallet yielded a little over $300 and a small bag of cocaine. I had no interest in his credit cards or ID, so once I removed the money and the little Baggie of coke, I shoved the wallet down deep into the trash, burying it under a drift of rough brown paper towels.

Later, when I was sure Desire was in the back restocking her ice, I slipped the plastic bag of cocaine into Joey's palm as a thank-you. The next time I saw him, his eyes were red and glassy and he was smiling and moving as jerkily and awkwardly as a mechanical toy, and I was glad that we were both on the same vibe, letting our good times roll.

Conclusion
Sealing the Deal

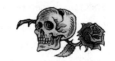

"Rusty Cage"— Soundgarden

When I first started stripping I thought it was the greatest, coolest job on earth. I felt like a special, chosen person, a girl so pretty and smart I could make money using only my wits and my courage and my body, trusting my instincts and accruing knowledge in a steep learning curve that was both exhausting and exhilarating. Then, right when I was in the thick of it, peeling my boundaries back in excruciating little slices, I began to suspect sex work was the worst, ugliest job ever, kind of like being a public toilet—a dreary, scary trudge of humiliation and disgust, leavened only by the company of other special, chosen women in the same boat.

The truth is that there are parts of this industry I love and parts of it that make me sick. My relationship with my work is complicated—sometimes I feel like the same pretty, smart girl I was ten years ago; other times I feel bitter and old and hateful. Either way, the adult industry welcomes me back every time I come knocking on the door looking for a place to stay and a way to earn my living. Going home feels warm and safe because I know I belong here with the women I love, in an industry I know better than anything else in the world. Maybe I'm just institutionalized, like the long-term convicts who get paroled and then immediately commit crimes just so they can go back to jail where things make sense and they know how everything works.

I kind of lost my mind in New Orleans—my moral compass was spinning without any magnetic reference, and I was lonely and horribly unhappy. Without my network of friends close at hand, I felt smaller and sadder and less important every day, as if I didn't count. I treated myself accordingly. It was as if I were torturing somebody I hated, except that person was me. And mostly I hated stage dancing—getting touched, getting drunk, stealing, lying. But at the same time there were moments when I'd pick my songs and go out and dance and feel like some kind of beautiful angel—light and free and happy—when I could just move to the music and feel my body as something fine and strong and vital that I loved with all my heart.

Hurricane Katrina came, and I evacuated New Orleans and went back to Seattle. By the time the hurricane came, I was so spun out by working at Fancy's that it was a relief to leave the city of rivers, lakes, and levees. I was one of the very, very lucky ones who got out pretty easily. I had nothing to lose and hadn't brought much, so when it was time to go, I evacuated to Little Rock, Arkansas, and flew home from there, paying for my plane ticket with a wad of twenties and fifties I'd made doing private shows at Fancy's.

Now I'm back in my hometown—Seattle—sleeping in a friend's spare room. He needs me out in a month, and I have no idea where I'm going to go then. I have a couch to crash on with a friend in Portland. Maybe I'll go down there, or maybe I'll try to rent a room here—I don't know. I know that wherever I go, there will be some little shack on the outskirts of town where men go to look at women's bodies, that I can walk into with my costumes and my makeup in a backpack and get a job and it'll be pretty much the same thing I've been doing for the last ten years. I'm free—unattached, untethered—and I have a trade. When I think about people who can't just pick up and move at whim—the ones with houses, families, and place-based jobs—I feel as wild and free as I sometimes felt onstage at Fancy's, like a joyous bird flying straight up into the sky.

Since coming home to Seattle, I've lost weight—a lot, I think, judging from the way my clothes are fitting—because I'm not drinking every day the way I was when I worked at Fancy's, and I'm going to the gym and working out hard four or five times a week. I feel good at the gym—peaceful. I listen to music on my iPod and pull air into my lungs in deep, grateful draughts. As I run on the treadmill, I feel as clean and neutral as a part of the machine myself—cool and blameless, like metal or plastic. I love the gym. After I come home and shower, I write. My life has become quiet and simple—pared down. Everything I don't need has fallen away—or was washed away in the hurricane.

Sometimes I dream about a place of my own—a little apartment somewhere, clean and pretty, all mine. A couch, and maybe even a bed, too—something besides a futon tossed on the floor. But I don't know how to live any other way. Having a lot of stuff—*owning* a lot of stuff—seems dangerous to me. Hurricane Katrina showed me how easily stuff can be taken away and wrecked. I think of how nice it would be to sit on a couch I own, reading a book—and then in the very next second all I can think about is losing it all, or having to beg people to help me move my shit the next time I leave town, and I realize that I feel safer without an anchor.

I went to Butterscotch's new location on Pacific Highway a few days ago and asked the current manager for my old job back. Pac Highway is an ugly, barren crawl, studded with ramshackle fast food establishments and the occasional massage parlor—or "spa," in the local parlance. The new Butterscotch's fits in well there, looking as shabby as any of its neighbors, as if the old Butterscotch's had simply been excised from its old location and imported with every streak of dirt and missing paint chip intact. The picture window in front is covered with tacked-up fabric and aluminum foil, and the neon sign that hangs in front of the fabric—in full view to the big-rig truckers who plod wearily up and down Pac Highway—features rudimentary, balloon-size breasts covered in two tiny triangular bra cups. The glowing pink breasts remind me of the dangling leg on the sign above Fancy's Foxhole, and of the eager fox with hearts for eyes and a pawful of cash.

None of the girls I worked with ten years ago are there now—Viva's gone, Crystal's gone, and nobody left forwarding addresses or phone numbers because the last thing you want is your personal information on the wall of some strip club, available to any customer creepy enough to convince a new girl you would have wanted him to have it.

Unsurprisingly, working at Butterscotch's is exactly the same as it was ten years ago—I'm wearing the same costumes, doing the same poses, delivering the same dirty talk, and watching the same masturbating monkeys applying the same bottle of baby oil to their peenies. Everything's the same, except I'm older. I started working when I was twenty-four, and now I'm thirty-four. So much has happened in between the first day I walked into Butterscotch's a decade ago and now that I can't even think about it all at once—I have to break it down into little pieces and squint at them that way, then put those pieces away and look at new ones. This is the only way I can gradually get a sense of the whole picture. But getting the *information* of the picture is one thing; deciding what it means is another. I can say the information of the picture in a few sentences. But I've been writing about what it *means* for 323 pages now, and I don't feel any closer to being done than I did when I first started writing this book a year ago.

I was so young when I started at Butterscotch's, with my dozen identical pairs of white cotton panties and my unshaven legs and my ninety-nine-cent tube of red lipstick. I walked into the lobby and met the most beautiful woman in the world and asked her if I was too fat to strip. Three days later I watched a man masturbate for the very first time, ever.

And now I've seen everything. I can't think of a single sexual variation I haven't witnessed, talked about, or performed. I've seen thousands of penises, from little fleshy bumps of skin that resemble buttons to freakishly oversize schlongs so immense their owners will never experience normal penetrative intercourse and are doomed to lives of chronic, two-handed masturbation. I've burned men with cigarettes and bloodied noses for money. I've watched my customers cry, and I've absorbed their rage; I've been the catalyst for so many orgasms I suspect the sheer mass of ejaculate I've supervised would fill an Olympic-size swimming pool. Gross, I know, but when it's in little spurts here and there it doesn't seem so foul. And most of it was into washcloths or Kleenex or paper towels, anyway.

Ideally, this is the part of the book where I thank you for spending your time reading my story and give you some idea of where I'm at now, or maybe say something Huge and Meaningful about the sex industry as a whole, so later on when you're thinking about what this book was about you can know for sure where I stand on adult work and use that as a way to figure out where *you* stand on it. Other, better writers—people who write and talk about the sex industry for a living—all seem to have firm conclusions, some of which I agree with and others I don't. I would like to provide some kind of definite conclusion, but I swore when I started writing this book that I'd tell the truth, even when the truth was bad or confusing or even just disappointing. I'd love to end this book with some kind of rallying cry but I can't, because the whole thing is too complex to be reduced down into some big, dumb slogan.

The truth is that I love the industry for what it's given me. I've spent ten years moving my body for a living, on my own terms.

When I think about all the other jobs a young woman can get with no work experience and no education—food service, office work, retail—I know that if I were doing it all over again I'd pick the sex industry over those options every single time, even knowing exactly how ugly and soul-killing it can get. The truth is I'm not good at working for other people, and I'm sure as hell not good at being told what to do. It also turns out I'm a hard worker—I just need a huge amount of personal autonomy. With it, I can roll in filth and still feel better about myself than I ever felt wiping down tables or making coffee.

The truth is I've run my own business for ten years, and done well for myself. I've taken time off when I've needed it, I've traveled, I've had adventures, and I've met the most amazing women in the world. I'm thirty-four and I'm healthy and strong and beautiful, and I live in a body that isn't perfect by Hollywood standards but every day I look in the mirror and I love what I see.

Stripping has shown me again and again that women of all shapes, ages, sizes, and appearances can be beautiful, confident, and joyously physical. And that's not just "head" knowledge—I wear that knowledge deep in my bones like marrow, and that knowing will stay with me for the rest of my life. That's a gift I've received from the industry, one that I didn't even know I could ask for, one I didn't even know I wanted or needed—the knowledge that it's just as valid to be of the body as it is to be of the mind. Dancing—moving your body, exercising, delighting in the purely physical—can be just as illuminating as reading. Now I make time for both.

When I talk to women who have never stripped and hear how they put themselves down and talk so mean about their own lovely, healthy bodies—whatever size they are, whatever shape they're in—it makes me wish that all women would try putting on sexy outfits and dancing to music they like—even if it's just in their own bedrooms, for their own pleasure. Maybe that would be a tiny little nudge toward a better world—one in which women accepted and celebrated themselves.

I'm not trying to soft-pedal the bad stuff inherent in the adult industry, though. What about the feelings of rage and hatred? What about the distrust? What about the humiliation of shaking your ass in some slob's face to make a few crumpled-up dollars that he'll try to shove into your pussy if you don't watch him like a hawk? What about the parts of the sex industry that aren't so *empowering,* like when you're broke and you let a customer come on your tits for $100 because you're just so fucking tired of saying no, and enforcing boundaries when all you really want to do is disconnect from your body and get the job done? What about the fact that the sex industry is basically predicated on a sexist fantasy of female submission to patriarchal authority, if you want to get all collegey about it? How can I call myself a feminist and do the work I do? How does doing this kind of work bring on the revolution, sister?

I wish I had better answers. It's true that I could have spent the past ten years working fifty hours a week just to pay my bills and keep a roof over my head, but I spent ten years working for myself instead—taking walks, going to museums, taking naps, and writing every day. Without a doubt, aspects of my work give me nightmares to this day—occurrences that even years later I remember, and the remembering makes me weep. I have frequent bad dreams about customers grabbing me, coming on me, raping me, hurting me—nightmares where I try to fight and my blows land softly and in slow motion, as if my fists were down pillows, and the customers laugh at me and continue to take what they want. Those dreams wake me up, and sometimes I can't get back to sleep. I also don't react well to being grabbed from behind, or to people who wave their hands in my face. Panic and rage are fairly close to the surface of my skin after working so long in a physically dangerous profession where any lapse of vigilance could result in assault or disease. The most unforgivable aspect of the sex industry is the fact that women are expected to assume physical risk for their customers' pleasure.

But my main problem with the adult industry is simply this: When we take part in it, we increase our alienation from each other. We become objects to each other, whether we're cash-vending objects or pleasure-vending objects. We take something as beautiful and communicative as sexual ecstasy and we commodify it, and in doing so we destroy everything that it stands for. We're not making love. As sex workers we're performing acts that we'd rather not be performing, with people we don't care about, because it's better than starving or working in a labor system that doesn't meet our needs. Or if we're customers, we're buying a poor semblance of affection that's so transparently false it bears almost no similarity to anything done in the spirit of honest love—and we know it, but we still seek out that kind of sexual service because it's easier or less frightening than trying to obtain the real thing.

And who gets what she or he really wants in any of these transactions? How much money is enough? What kind of sexual thrill is intense enough to justify what we're losing?

I think that even in the best possible transactions—those in which neither party is harmed, the vendor receives a large amount of money, and the client receives exemplary service—everyone's getting ripped off, because we're taking an act that is essentially about human communication and caring, and perverting it into something that's impersonal at best, and full of contempt and hatred at worst. The more we become accustomed to buying and selling sexual service, the less space we permit in our lives for the real thing. And the less we care about other people, the colder and more hostile the world becomes.

I'm not trying to pretend that I haven't been part of the problem. Ten years ago I became an adult entertainer as a way to make money on my own terms—then, once I began to reflect on my work, I continued because I was writing, and because I was being turned to by others as an expert in my field. I figured you can't report on a war if you don't get right down into the trenches, and so I stayed. I still think I made the right decision—to stay, and to witness. Because whether or not you vend or buy adult service, all of us live in a society that supports the sex industry as a massive, multibillion-dollar concern. Do we like it the way it is? Or would we like to make some changes to it, or even tear it down entirely and start something new and completely different?

We can, after all—it belongs to every single one of us. It's *ours*.

"s(AINT)"— Marilyn Manson

I am in the dungeon at Butterscotch's, with a client. He stands stolidly, his hands bound behind his back with soft white cotton rope. He is nude, with a rubber band cruelly constricting the base of his small, soft cock. The pillowcase over his head—and the way he stands passively, waiting for further instruction—lends him an undeniable resemblance to the emblematic Abu Ghraib prisoner posed on a box with wires running from his fingertips.

"You little whore," I say. "Do you know what happens to whores?" I am bluffing—I have no specific plans for punishment. I figure I can hit him with a paddle for a while, or possibly clamp his nipples. Most domination clients are just happy to be the center of attention, to be spoken to, and to have someone make plans that will come to fruition on their bodies.

My customer whimpers. "No, ma'am," he says. His cock twitches in interest.

I seize a wooden paddle from its hook on the wall of the dungeon and use it to spank the lower arcs of my client's buttocks, careful to avoid his bound hands. I spank lightly—really, I'm only tapping him. If I'd planned the session a little better, I would have tied his hands in front, leaving his ass open to punishment. But none of it really matters. He only has ten minutes of his session time left anyway. I'll spank him for a while, then untie him and let him jerk off, and then we'll be done.

"Oh, Mistress," he moans. "Oh, have mercy on your little whore."

I laugh. "Never!" I say. I'm Snidely Whiplash in a G-string. I keep tapping his bottom lightly as he squirms in delight. *This could be worse,* I think. He's happy, the scene is easy, and—it feels good to be home.

Acknowledgments

Everything that sucks in this book is my fault.

Everything that rocks is due to the diabolical perfectionism of my editor, Ms. Brooke Warner. Miss B: *Thank you,* with all my heart.

Thank you to my LiveJournal friends—you know who you are. Thanks for cheering me on and for sending me clothes, food, money, and treats when I needed them desperately. There's absolutely no way this book would even exist without you. (Go here to read my blog: markedformetal.livejournal.com.)

Thank you to my brother Noah Aloysius Birnel—for cooking me delicious food, for standing up for me, and for always being proud of me. You're a good man and I love you, Noah. Now hurry up and make me an auntie.

And thank you, once more, to the working girls who've inspired me and shown me what it means to be brilliant, complicated, brave, loving women: Noelle. Tara/Daisy. Klaudia. Cake. Evelyn. Anastasia. Gina. Lydia. Tamara. Dara and Jolie. Diana/Daphne. Stella. Orchid. Athena.

I am honored to know and love you all.

Acknowledgments

About the Author

Sarah Katherine Lewis is thirty-four years old and has been working in the sex industry for more than a decade, in Seattle, Portland, and New Orleans. She's worked as a stripper, a lingerie model, a phone sex operator, a dominatrix, a body worker, a live-stream adult web performer, an XXX model, and a porn star. Lewis was featured on NPR reading a piece from her blog, and will appear in the upcoming documentary film *Fantasies Matter: Pornography, Sexualities, and Relationships.*

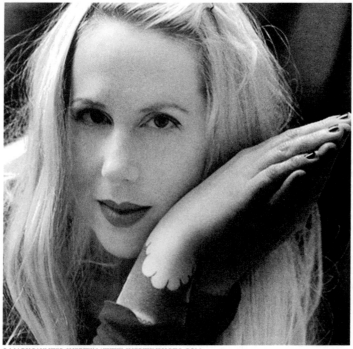

© MARY PAYNTER SHERWIN / WWW.SHERWINPHOTO.COM

Selected Titles from Seal Press

For more than thirty years, Seal Press has published groundbreaking books. By women. For women. Visit our website at www.sealpress.com.

Pissed Off: On Women and Anger by Spike Gillespie. $14.95, 1-58005-162-6. An amped up and personal self-help book that encourages women to go ahead and use that middle finger without being closed off to the notion of forgiveness.

Bare: The Naked Truth About Stripping by Elisabeth Eaves. $14.95, 1-58005-121-9. A closer look at the way sexuality is viewed in our culture: what, if anything, constitutes "normal" desire and the ethics of swapping money—or anything else—for sex.

Body Outlaws: Rewriting the Rules of Beauty and Body Image edited by Ophira Edut, foreward by Rebecca Walker. $15.95, 1-58005-075. Filled with honesty and humor, this groundbreaking anthology offers stories by women who have chosen to ignore, subvert, or redefine the dominate beauty standard in order to feel at home in their bodies.

Cunt: A Declaration of Independence by Inga Muscio. $14.95, 1-58005-075-1. "An insightful, sisterly, and entertaining exploration of the word and the part of the body it so bluntly defines. Ms. Muscio muses, reminisces, pokes into history and emerges with suggestions for the understanding of—and reconciliation with—what it means to have a cunt."—Roberta Gregory, author of *Naughty Bitch*

Without a Net: The Female Experience of Growing Up Working Class by Michelle Tea. $14.95, 1-58005-103-0. A collection of essays "so raw, so fresh, and so riveting that I read them compulsively, with one hand alternately covering my mouth, my heart, and my stomach, while the other hand turned the page. *Without a Net* is an important book for any woman who's grown up—or is growing up—in America."—Vendela Vida, *And Now You Can Go*

Listen Up: Voices from the Next Feminist Generation edited by Barbara ᵈlen. $16.95, 1-58005-054-9. A collection of eight essays featuring ᵉs of today's young feminists on racism, sexuality, identity, AIDS, ᵒn, abortion, and much more.